Psychiatry

PreTest®
Self-Assessment
and Review

Psychiatry

PreTest®
Self-Assessment
and Review

Sixth Edition

Sherwyn M. Woods, M.D., Ph.D.

Professor of Psychiatry
Director, Student Psychiatric Health Service
Director, Psychoanalytic Education
University of Southern California School of Medicine
Los Angeles County/USC Medical Center
Los Angeles, California

McGraw-Hill, Inc.
Health Professions Division/PreTest® Series

New York	St. Louis	San Francisco	Auckland
Bogotá	Caracas	Lisbon	London	Madrid
Mexico	Milan	Montreal	New Delhi	Paris
San Juan	Singapore	Sydney	Tokyo	Toronto

Psychiatry: PreTest® Self-Assessment and Review
International Edition 1991.

1 2 3 4 5 6 7 8 9 0 AP PMP 9 5 4 3 2 1

ISBN 0-07-051986-2

The editors were Gail Gavert and Bruce MacGregor.
The production supervisor was Clara B. Stanley.
This book was set in Times Roman by R.J. Landi
Book Production.

Library of Congress Cataloging-in-Publication Data

Psychiatry : PreTest self-assessment and review —
edited by Sherwyn M. Woods

   p. cm.
  Includes bibliographical references.
  ISBN 0-07-051986-2 :
  1. Psychiatry — Examinations, questions, etc. I. Woods,
Sherwyn M.
  [DNLM: 1. Psychiatry — examinations, questions. WM 18 P978]
RC457.P78 1991
616.89'0076 — dc20
DNLM/DLC
for Library of Congress   90-13710
                CIP

When ordering this title, use ISBN 0-07-112776-3.

Printed in Singapore.

Contents

Preface

This sixth edition of *Psychiatry: PreTest® Self-Assessment and Review* has been extensively revised. The field of psychiatry has been covered in greater depth and breadth. The questions and explanations are consistent with the terminology and definitions employed by the revised third edition of the *Diagnostic and Statistical Manual* of the American Psychiatric Association. Also, the number of K-type questions has been reduced in keeping with the intentions of the National Board of Medical Examiners. The references have been updated, and all questions are referenced to standard textbooks or other major resource books that are readily available in most libraries.

I would like to express special gratitude to my wife, Nancy Bricard Woods, for her encouragement, patience, and support. I am also deeply appreciative of the assistance of all those who were so helpful in the preparation of this manuscript, especially my secretary, Mary Jane Costello.

Sherwyn M. Woods, M.D., Ph.D.

Preface

Introduction

Psychiatry: PreTest® Self-Assessment and Review, 6th Ed., has been designed to provide medical students, psychiatric residents, psychiatrists, mental health professionals, and international medical graduates with a comprehensive and convenient instrument for self-assessment and review within the field of psychiatry. The 500 questions provided have been designed to parallel the topics, format, and degree of difficulty of the questions contained in the Comprehensive Part II of the National Board of Medical Examiners examinations and the Foreign Medical Graduate Examination in the Medical Sciences (FMGEMS). They will continue to be a useful study tool for Steps 2 and 3 of the United States Medical Licensing Examination (USMLE). The questions are also of a style and variety that should prove useful to those preparing for the certification examinations of the American Board of Psychiatry and Neurology.

Each question in this book is accompanied by an answer, a paragraph explanation, and a specific page reference to a textbook or major resource. These books and standard textbooks have been carefully selected for their educational excellence and ready availability in most libraries. A bibliography that lists all the sources used in this book follows the last chapter.

One effective way to use this book is to allow yourself one minute to answer each question in a given chapter, marking your answer beside each question. By following this suggestion, you will be approximating the time limits imposed by the examinations previously mentioned.

Since there are few absolutes in clinical practice, remember to simply choose the best possible answer. There are no "trick" questions intended. Rather, each has been designed to address a significant topical area. All questions apply to the evaluation and treatment of adults, unless children or adolescents are specifically mentioned.

When you have finished answering the questions in a chapter, you should then spend as much time as you need to verify your answers and carefully read the explanations. You should read every explanation, but pay special attention to the questions you answered incorrectly. Each explanation has been designed to reinforce and supplement the information being tested by each question. When you identify an important gap in your fund of knowledge, or if you simply need more information about the topic, you should consult and study the references indicated.

Evaluation, Assessment, and Diagnosis

DIRECTIONS: Each question below contains five suggested responses. Select the one best response to each question.

1. The most frequent indication for psychological testing in clinical psychiatry is

(A) to determine the correct dosage of medication
(B) to determine the most effective psychotherapeutic style
(C) to assist when there is uncertainty about the diagnosis
(D) to assist in determining the length of treatment
(E) to assist in generating clinical impressions

2. Evaluation of thyroid function may be particularly helpful in the diagnosis and treatment of which of the following conditions?

(A) Phobic disorder
(B) Schizotypal personality disorder
(C) Major depression
(D) Schizophrenia
(E) None of the above

3. While genetic factors are believed to play a role in the etiology of many psychiatric disorders, studies have shown the most frequently positive family history in

(A) generalized anxiety disorder
(B) bipolar disorder
(C) social phobia
(D) panic disorder
(E) somatoform disorder

4. Brain-imaging techniques, such as computed tomography (CT), would be most useful in evaluating

(A) bipolar disorder
(B) schizophrenia
(C) panic disorder
(D) Alzheimer dementia
(E) sleep apnea

5. All the following are projective tests EXCEPT

(A) Rorschach
(B) Thematic Apperception Test
(C) Zung
(D) draw a human figure
(E) sentence completion

6. The intelligence quotient (IQ) is best described as a measure of

(A) innate cognitive endowment
(B) future cognitive potential
(C) environmentally determined cognitive skill
(D) present functional cognitive ability
(E) learned verbal skills

7. Which of the following descriptions is true regarding persons who are at particular risk to commit suicide?

(A) They rarely communicate their intent
(B) They seldom have close family members who died by suicide
(C) They are almost always psychotic
(D) They rarely have a history of previous suicide attempts
(E) None of the above

8. A delusion can best be defined as a

(A) false belief that meets specific psychological needs
(B) perceptual misrepresentation of a sensory image
(C) perceptual representation of a sound or object not actually present
(D) viewpoint able to be changed when convincing evidence to the contrary is presented
(E) dissociative reaction

9. In the United States the statistical suicide rate is higher in persons who are

(A) male rather than female
(B) single rather than divorced
(C) black rather than white
(D) married rather than widowed
(E) young rather than old

10. A 7-year-old girl hospitalized for a tonsillectomy awakens and cries out in fright that a "big bear" is in her room. She is relieved when a nurse, responding to her cry, enters the room and turns on the light, revealing the bear to be an armchair covered with a coat. This experience would be an example of

(A) a delusion
(B) a hallucination
(C) an illusion
(D) déjà vu
(E) dissociative reaction

11. Calculation of an IQ score requires knowledge of an examinee's

(A) mental age and educational level
(B) chronologic age and educational level
(C) mental age and chronologic age
(D) mental age, chronologic age, and educational level
(E) mental age and psychiatric history

12. An 18-year-old woman, previously in good health, seeks help at an emergency room for lightheadedness, headaches, and nausea. She appears anxious and is tremulous, sweating, and breathing heavily. While waiting to see a physician, she begins to complain of tingling around her mouth and in her fingertips. The physician should first

(A) ask her to breathe into a paper bag
(B) order immediate intravenous infusion of 50 mL of 50% glucose solution
(C) arrange for a brain scan
(D) conduct an amobarbital interview
(E) draw a blood sample to evaluate blood alcohol concentration

Questions 13–14

As a part of the mental status examination, an interviewee is asked for the meaning of the proverb "People in glass houses should not throw stones." The person replies, "They will break the windows."

13. This response is an example of

(A) idiosyncratic thinking
(B) concrete thinking
(C) bizarre ideation
(D) loose associations
(E) none of the above

14. Patients who interpret proverbs in this way most often have a diagnosis of

(A) dysthymia
(B) paranoid personality disorder
(C) panic disorder
(D) passive aggressive personality disorder
(E) schizophrenia

15. Feelings about an interviewee may be aroused in an interviewer by the interviewee's resemblance to someone in the interviewer's past. This is an example of

(A) displacement
(B) projection
(C) illusion
(D) countertransference
(E) identification

16. The Minnesota Multiphasic Personality Inventory (MMPI) is

(A) a subjective test
(B) a projective test
(C) an intelligence test
(D) a personality test
(E) a special aptitude test

17. Psychiatric rating scales that have been developed to evaluate symptoms and psychopathology include all the following EXCEPT

(A) Hamilton Rating Scale for Depression (Hamilton)
(B) Mental Status Examination Record (MSER)
(C) Present State Examination (PSE)
(D) Brief Psychiatric Rating Scale (BPRS)
(E) Social Adjustment Scale (SAS)

18. A 69-year-old man is suspected of having an acute onset of multiple small cerebral infarcts. The finding on mental status examination that would be most supportive of this diagnosis is

(A) a change in cognitive functioning
(B) depressed mood
(C) inappropriate affect
(D) delusional thinking
(E) anxiety

19. In documenting the mental status examination, all the following are reported EXCEPT

(A) appearance
(B) behavior
(C) speech
(D) sleep pattern
(E) mood and affect

Questions 20–21

The format for the reporting of diagnoses detailed by the *Diagnostic and Statistical Manual of the American Psychiatric Association (DSM III-R)* is multiaxial. Each case is assessed along several axes, each of which is descriptive of a different class of information.

20. The presence of a personality disorder would be reported on

(A) axis I
(B) axis II
(C) axis III
(D) axis IV
(E) axis V

21. A physical illness that was relevant to either diagnosis or management would be reported on

(A) axis I
(B) axis II
(C) axis III
(D) axis IV
(E) axis V

22. A person sitting alone and behaving as if listening intently suddenly begins to nod and mutter aloud. This person most likely is experiencing

(A) a delusion
(B) an illusion
(C) a hallucination
(D) an idea of reference
(E) a flight of ideas

23. The Bender-Gestalt test is most often used in the diagnostic assessment of

(A) personality disorders
(B) organic disorders
(C) mood disorders
(D) anxiety disorders
(E) sleep disorders

DIRECTIONS: Each question below contains four suggested responses of which **one or more** is correct. Select

A	if	**1, 2, and 3**	are correct
B	if	**1 and 3**	are correct
C	if	**2 and 4**	are correct
D	if	**4**	is correct
E	if	**1, 2, 3, and 4**	are correct

24. When there is a possible diagnosis of sleep apnea, it is particularly important to take a history from the spouse

(1) to determine whether the patient snores
(2) to evaluate the presence of marital discord
(3) to confirm the patient's daytime sleepiness
(4) to evaluate the spouse's typical sleep pattern

25. Psychological assessment can provide useful data in which of the following areas?

(1) Symptom severity and change
(2) Cognitive functioning
(3) Personality dynamics
(4) Psychiatric research

26. A 40-year-old woman complains of fatigue, difficulty sleeping, and vague aches and pains and is preoccupied with her physical health. This clinical picture can suggest the presence of

(1) an occult carcinoma
(2) an endocrinopathy
(3) influenza
(4) depression

27. Diagnostic evaluation of a child with suspected mental retardation would include

(1) careful physical examination
(2) neurologic examination
(3) examination of urine and blood for metabolic disorders
(4) psychological testing

28. Assessment of psychiatric disorders according to the format detailed in the revised third edition of *Diagnostic and Statistical Manual of Mental Disorders (DSM III-R)* would include a statement or description of

(1) clinical diagnosis
(2) etiology
(3) best level of functioning in the last 12 months
(4) family history of mental illness

29. In psychiatry the electroencephalogram (EEG) has particular usefulness in the diagnosis of

(1) panic disorder
(2) delirium
(3) schizophrenia
(4) episodic disorders such as rage reactions

30. Interpretation of responses to the Rorschach test may be used to help

(1) diagnose schizophrenia
(2) describe personality strengths
(3) reveal capacity for interpersonal relationships
(4) obtain an IQ measurement

31. In narcolepsy, the polysomnographic recording typically shows

(1) an absence of REM sleep in midcycle
(2) anoxia
(3) spike and wave EEG recording
(4) an REM period shortly after sleep onset

DIRECTIONS: Each group of questions below consists of lettered headings followed by a set of numbered items. For each numbered item select the **one** lettered heading with which it is **most** closely associated. Each lettered heading may be used **once, more than once, or not at all.**

Questions 32–36

Match the following.

(A) Memory impairment
(B) Thought broadcasting
(C) Recurrent self-damaging acts
(D) Perfectionism
(E) Pathologic jealousy

32. Paranoid personality disorder

33. Borderline personality disorder

34. Dementia

35. Schizophrenia

36. Obsessive compulsive personality disorder

Questions 37–40

Match the following.

(A) Prevalence
(B) Incidence
(C) Validity
(D) Primary prevention
(E) Secondary prevention

37. Early case finding and treatment to minimize duration of illness and to prevent permanent disability

38. The proportion of a population affected by a disorder at a given time

39. The proportion of a population that becomes affected by a disorder for the first time in a given period of time

40. Attempting to discover and eliminate the causes of mental illness

Questions 41–44

Match the following.

(A) Magical thinking
(B) Blocking
(C) Looseness of associations
(D) Derealization
(E) Depersonalization

41. Discontinuous and illogical stream of thoughts

42. A belief that thought alone can result in the accomplishment of certain wishes or activities

43. Sudden cessation of thinking in the middle of a discussion or sentence

44. The feeling that one is standing apart from oneself and observing one's own actions

DIRECTIONS: The group of questions below consists of four lettered headings followed by a set of numbered items. For each numbered item select

A	if the item is associated with	(A) only
B	if the item is associated with	(B) only
C	if the item is associated with	both (A) and (B)
D	if the item is associated with	neither (A) nor (B)

Each lettered heading may be used once, more than once, or not at all.

Questions 45–47

(A) Reliability
(B) Validity
(C) Both
(D) Neither

45. A measure of a test's ability to actually assess what it claims to

46. A measure of a test's reproducibility

47. A measure of the ability of a test's results to represent more than chance

Evaluation, Assessment, and Diagnosis

Answers

1.   **The answer is C.** *(Michels, vol 1, chap 7, p 3.)* The most frequent reason for the use of psychological testing in a clinical psychiatric setting is assisting when there is uncertainty about diagnosis. Unlike semistructured interviews that generate broad clinical impressions, psychological testing yields specific, comparable information about diagnosis and severity of symptoms. It is not useful in determining medications or dosages or length of treatment. No diagnosis should be made strictly on the results of testing, but these results are useful when confronting difficult diagnostic problems.

2.   **The answer is C.** *(Hales, pp 315–320.)* Many of the signs and symptoms of hypothyroidism are similar to those seen in major depression, and thus thyroid testing is an important part of the differential diagnostic process. Some degree of hypothyroidism has been found in a significant percentage of both inpatients and outpatients being treated for depression. Thyroid testing should definitely be considered when depressed patients complain of a lack of energy, have symptoms or a family history of thyroid disorder, or fail to respond to antidepressant medication.

3.   **The answer is B.** *(Kaplan, ed 5. pp 879–887.)* There has been an ever-increasing interest in elucidating the genetic issues involved in predisposition to psychiatric disorders. Studies have shown that genetic factors are probably present in a wide variety of illnesses, including most of the anxiety disorders. Such studies are often difficult to interpret because of the special strategies needed to control for psychosocial factors that may be perpetuated in families. Extensive twin and adoptive studies have provided the best evidence for an important genetic factor in the etiology of mood disorders, including bipolar, and in schizophrenia. A positive family history is particularly common in these two illnesses.

4.   **The answer is D.** *(Kaplan, ed 5. pp 92–104.)* Brain-imaging techniques include x-ray, computed tomography (CT), emission tomography, nuclear magnetic resonance imaging (MRI), and positron emission tomography (PET). These techniques are widely employed in research studies of virtually all psychiatric conditions, but in most instances the findings do not have major diagnostic value. In the dementias, however, abnormalities on CT scan are present in a large number of

patients, including those with dementias of the Alzheimer type. The findings are not speci̇ ̇ enough to differentiate Alzheimer dementia from other senile dementias, or even at times from normal controls. The findings might be helpful in distinguishing dementia from the "pseudodementia" that may accompany severe depression.

5.   The answer is C. *(Michels, vol 1, chap 7, pp 8-9.)* Projective tests are standardized assessments using unstructured situations that allow for a patient's personality dynamics and style to emerge in a nonthreatening way. The Rorschach inkblot test is one of the best known; however, the Thematic Apperception Test, draw a figure, and sentence completion test are also widely used and effective. The Zung is a test used for depression. It is a symptom-oriented self-assessment instrument that gathers data and is not projective in nature.

6.   The answer is D. *(Kaplan, ed 5. pp 497-499.)* Intelligence quotient (IQ) is a measure of a person's ability to function cognitively at the time of testing. Excessive fatigue, psychosis, and brain damage are three factors that can change a person's ability to function and thus affect IQ measurement. Neither environmental nor innate (genetic) origins of intelligence are measured directly by the IQ test. Skilled interpreters, however, can infer from the responses to an intelligence test how these and other factors, including poor motivation and poor rapport with an examiner, might have affected the IQ score.

7.   The answer is E. *(Kaplan, ed 5. pp 1414-1427.)* The psychiatric history is of considerable usefulness in evaluating risk for suicide. Patients at particular risk are more likely to have a history of psychiatric disorder (especially depression) and family members who have committed suicide. A past suicide attempt is perhaps the best predictor of increased risk. While psychosis is a definite risk factor, the majority of successful suicides occur in persons who are not psychotic. Most commonly, patients who commit suicide have directly or subtly communicated their intent prior to the act.

8.   The answer is A. *(Michels, vol 1, chap 68, p 1; vol 2, chap 87, p 1.)* A delusion is a false belief that is not supported by fact and cannot be challenged successfully by logic or reason. Delusions are not randomly selected but rather develop as a defense against or support for specific thoughts or experiences; consequently, delusional thinking is said to be under the control of emotional, not rational, forces. What might be viewed as delusional to members of one social or cultural group may not be viewed as such by members of a widely divergent culture or social system.

9.   The answer is A. *(Kaplan, ed 5. pp 1414-1415.)* In the United States it has been found that suicide rates increase with increasing age, and at all ages males commit suicide more often than females in ratios that range from 2:1 to 7:1.

Married persons have the lowest suicide rate, with singles twice as apt, and widowed persons five times more likely to kill themselves. Blacks have a lower suicide rate than whites, and Jews and Catholics a lower rate than Protestants.

10. The answer is C. *(Michels, vol 1, chap 68, p 1.)* An illusion is a misinterpretation of an actual sensory stimulus. A person's emotional state and personality needs can play an important role in determining the presence and type of an illusion. For example, perhaps the girl described in the question thought she saw a bear in her room because the hospital is a frightening, hostile environment for her. Systemic disease states associated with confusion (certain types of poisoning, for instance) also can produce misperceptions of sensory images by interfering with proper functioning of the brain.

11. The answer is C. *(Michels, vol 2, chap 21, p 4.)* IQ scores are determined by taking the ratio of mental age to chronologic age and multiplying by 100. This system of calculating the IQ was developed by W. L. Stern. The IQ is an indicator of relative brightness and can be used to compare children of different ages when mental age continues to increase in proportion to chronologic age.

12. The answer is A. *(Kaplan, ed 5. pp 1198–1199.)* The woman described in the question likely is experiencing a hyperventilation syndrome. Hyperventilation, which commonly is associated with acute anxiety reactions, causes excessive loss of carbon dioxide and, as a result, leads to respiratory alkalosis. As blood pH rises ionization of calcium decreases, and clinical signs of tetany, such as painful muscle spasms in the hands, can become manifest. Other symptoms of hyperventilation include lightheadedness, headache, nausea, and tingling around the mouth and in the fingers and toes. Breathing into a paper bag reverses the symptoms because the reinspired air has a higher concentration of carbon dioxide than does normal air.

13–14. The answers are: 13-B, 14-E. *(Kaplan, ed 5. pp 561–562.)* Part of the task of the mental status examination is to examine the patient for the presence of a thought disorder. An inability to form abstract concepts, illustrated by literalmindedness, is demonstrated by the concrete interpretation of proverbs. It is a form of thought disorder called *concrete thinking.* Generally several proverbs are asked of the patient in order to make the determination. Concrete thinking is seen particularly in patients with organic brain disorder, and also in patients with schizophrenia. It is definitely not a part of the clinical picture in personality disorders or in the neuroses.

15. The answer is D. *(Michels, vol 3, chap 36, pp 9–10.)* When feelings an interviewer develops for an interviewee are based on irrational, unconscious factors—for example, the interviewee's resemblance to someone in the interviewer's past—countertransference is said to be in operation. Sometimes these feelings can be positive; other times, negative. Although physicians and other psychotherapists are apt to like some patients more than others, inordinate feelings of anger or antagonism toward certain patients should prompt a search for what it is about the patient that is bothersome. The problems may relate more to an unresolved conflict within the interviewer than to the actual personality of the interviewee.

16.   The answer is D. *(Michels, vol 1, chap 7, p 5; vol 1, chap 15, p 5.)* The Minnesota Multiphasic Personality Inventory (MMPI) is a questionnaire designed to measure various dimensions of personality. Examination of the responses rates the test subject according to nine clinical scales. Because it has been administered to large numbers of normal and emotionally disturbed subjects, considerable normative data are available. It can be administered to a large group of persons at one time and scored by computer.

17.   The answer is E. *(Kaplan, ed 5. pp 534-552.)* Psychiatric rating scales have been developed to evaluate response to treatment in a variety of dimensions. They differ in a variety of ways, including their administration, content, and validity. The Social Adjustment Scale is oriented toward assessment of social contacts as opposed to specific psychiatric symptoms. The Hamilton Rating Scale for Depression was first published in 1960 and is the most widely used instrument by which interviewers rate and assess depression. The MSER is a computer-coded instrument that details the patient's symptomatology and current mental status. The BPRS, published by Overall and Gorham in 1962, is a commonly used research instrument that allows for the rating of a variety of dimensions of psychopathology.

18.   The answer is A. *(Hales, pp 4-15.)* The possibility of an acute organic brain disorder mandates a careful examination of cognitive function. Acute conditions would be associated with a determination that the patient's cognitive ability had changed. For example, poor calculation skills in a person who had been a functioning accountant would be far more significant than the same findings in someone with a long history of poor school performance. It is the assessment of *change* in cognitive function, rather than the specific cognitive disturbance, that is most crucial to a diagnosis of acute organic brain disorder. This is what helps the clinician to differentiate memory or other cognitive deficits of recent onset from those which are long standing.

19.   The answer is D. *(Kaplan, ed 5. pp 145-147, 463-465.)* The mental status examination has a standard format. Sleep pattern is important to assess in taking a psychiatric history, but it is not part of the written mental status examination. A cogent description of appearance, behavior, speech, mood, and affect is required.

20-21.   The answers are: 20-B, 21-C. *(American Psychiatric Association, ed 3-R. pp 15-17.)* Axis I and axis II constitute the entire classification of mental disorders as defined by *DSM III-R*. Axis I consists of the clinical syndromes. Axis II lists both developmental disorders and personality disorders and can also be used to indicate specific personality traits or the habitual use of particular defense mechanisms. Multiple diagnoses can be recorded on both axis I and axis II. Axis III is used to record any current medical condition, physical disorder, or physical condition relevant to understanding or managing the case. So-called soft neurologic signs could be included here. Multiple diagnoses are permitted on this axis. Using these axes, a patient with depression might be recorded as follows: axis I—major depression, recurrent; axis II—narcissistic personality disorder; axis III—hypothyroidism.

22.   The answer is C. *(Kaplan, ed 5. pp 570-572.)* A hallucination is the perception of a stimulus when, in fact, no sensory stimulus is present. Hallucinations can be auditory, visual, tactile, gustatory, olfactory, or kinesthetic. Auditory hallucinations are most commonly associated with psychotic illness, whereas visual, tactile, gustatory, and olfactory hallucinations are associated with neurologic disorders.

23.   The answer is B. *(Kaplan, ed 5. p 508.)* The Bender-Gestalt test is one of visual motor function and is used in both children and adults. It is one of the well-known but older tests used to determine the possible presence of an organic brain disorder. The test consists of asking the patient to copy nine figures. It has limited value and has been largely replaced by more sophisticated measurements.

24.   The answer is B (1, 3). *(Talbott, pp 746-747.)* In obstructive sleep apnea, one of the most common clinical findings is loud snoring. The patient may be unaware of this except from the description of others. These patients often thrash about in their sleep, gasp at the end of a period of apnea, and on occasion may wet the bed. The symptoms are very disruptive to the sleep of others, and thus an objective history may reveal information the patient is unable to provide.

25.   The answer is E (all). *(Michels, vol 1, chap 7, p 1.)* Psychological assessment, which can be done with a wide variety of instruments, provides quantitative data in a variety of areas including symptom severity, cognitive functioning, and personality dynamics. Choosing the appropriate test is crucial and requires an understanding of the instrument and its limitations. Owing to the standardization of these tests, they are particularly useful in conducting psychiatric research.

26.   The answer is E (all). *(Kaplan, ed 5. pp 896-902.)* The presence of vague aches and pains and preoccupation with somatic complaints can point to a diagnosis of depression. Often, depressed patients present clinically with a particular physical symptom, such as backache, and not with psychological disturbances. However, depressive syndromes also can be associated with medical conditions, such as occult malignancies, or be a manifestation of an endocrinopathy—particularly Cushing's syndrome, hypothyroidism, and hyperparathyroidism. Viral diseases, especially during their incubation and convalescent stages, also can produce a depressive syndrome. Thus, patients presenting with the signs and symptoms of depression should receive a thorough medical evaluation.

27.   The answer is E (all). *(Kaplan, ed 5. pp 1728–1730.)* A variety of conditions may simulate mental retardation. Careful diagnostic evaluation may reveal specific sensory handicaps, which may be mistaken for mental retardation. Chronic medical diseases can depress the child's functioning in several areas. Differential diagnostic expertise is required to rule out deafness or visual impairment in an infant or toddler. Speech deficits and cerebral palsy must be considered in differential diagnosis. Any neurologic disorder, including seizure disorders, may give an impression of mental retardation. The coexistence of severe behavioral manifestations of a childhood psychiatric disorder makes the evaluation very difficult.

28.   The answer is B (1, 3). *(American Psychiatric Association, ed 3-R pp 15–24.)* *Diagnostic and Statistical Manual of Mental Disorders*, revised third edition *(DSM III-R)*, attempts to categorize psychiatric disturbances according to a number of criteria. There is a separate "axis" to describe each of the following parameters: clinical diagnosis, personality diagnosis, associated medical conditions, severity of psychosocial stress, and best level of adaptive functioning currently and during the last year. This system is used to describe the clinical manifestations of a mental disorder and not how the disorder arose.

29.   The answer is C (2, 4). *(Kaplan, ed 5. pp 161–165, 625.)* The EEG is a very useful diagnostic tool in distinguishing delirium from functional psychosis and in evaluating episodic behavioral disorders. It may reveal organic pathology that is not demonstrable by other means, such as the CT scan. EEG abnormalities are not a usual finding in the neuroses or in schizophrenia.

30.   The answer is A (1, 2, 3). *(Kaplan, ed 5. p 483. Michels, vol 1, chap 7, p 7.)* The test devised by the Swiss psychiatrist Hermann Rorschach consists of a set of ten inkblots that serve as stimuli for association. It is a projective test because subjects are forced to demonstrate how they think and perceive by finding meaningful symbols or shapes in a formless design. Responses can be compared with responses made by normal persons and persons with known disorders. Responses to cards that usually appear to present human forms may illuminate interpersonal attitudes or personality traits. Poor form perception and idiosyncratic or peculiar associations are examples of the type of responses made by schizophrenic persons. The Rorschach test is not a test of intelligence.

31.   The answer is D (4). *(Talbott, pp 747–748.)* Patients with narcolepsy quite probably have a defect in REM inhibition. When sleep recordings are made, the patients typically show a sleep-onset REM period, or one that occurs very shortly after the onset of sleep. From 15 to 30 percent may also show some nocturnal myoclonus or sleep apnea.

32-36. The answers are: 32-E, 33-C, 34-A, 35-B, 36-D. *(American Psychiatric Association, ed 3-R, pp 103-107, 187-196, 337-338, 346-347, 354-356.)* The paranoid personality is characterized by litigiousness, expectation of harm, and guardedness. Because these patients question the loyalty of others, they may often experience pathologic jealousy. During severe stress, transient psychotic symptoms may occur, but these do not persist.

The borderline personality as defined by *DSM III-R* is characterized by emotional instability in a variety of areas including self-image. This results in unpredictable behavior that may be potentially self-damaging. Short-lived psychotic episodes have been described as micropsychotic. Delusional ideas that may occur are typically not bizarre.

Dementia typically interferes with social or occupational functioning because of significant memory impairment. Changes in personality and behavior may also occur. Reversibility of the memory impairment depends on the underlying cause. In most cases, however, short- and long-term memory deficits persist.

Schizophrenia is a major psychotic illness involving disturbance in psychologic processes. There is a deterioration in level of functioning during some phases of the illness. Characteristic bizarre delusions such as thought broadcasting are more common in patients with schizophrenia than in patients with other psychotic disorders.

Finally, the compulsive personality is often described as perfectionistic. The patient may be preoccupied with rules, details, and orders. However, difficulty with decision making may manifest itself as part of the clinical presentation. The behavior of the compulsive personality reflects the need for organization and an urge for self-control. Such a patient has been called the orderly, controlling type, and this personality configuration is similar to the so-called type A personality.

37-40. The answers are: 37-E, 38-A, 39-B, 40-D. *(Nicholi, pp 762-767, 783.)* All the terms listed in the question group are particularly common to psychiatric epidemiology. Prevalence studies in psychiatry are far more common than incidence studies. Prevalence equals the cases in the population divided by the total population (cases plus noncases). It is generally measured at a given point in time (point prevalence) or over a given period of time (period prevalence). It counts both old and new cases, in contrast to incidence, which is a measure of the number of new cases that occur in a specified period.

Validity refers to the accuracy and verifiability of a study. It is usually demonstrated by agreement between two attempts to measure the same issue by different methods.

Primary prevention represents the attempt to discover and then eliminate the causes of illness, while secondary prevention relates to early case finding and treatment to shorten the illness and prevent permanent disability. Tertiary prevention is involved with rehabilitation.

41-44. The answers are: 41-C, 42-A, 43-B, 44-E. *(Kaplan, ed 5. pp 471-474, 989.)* Looseness of associations refers to a string of thoughts that are disconnected in content and are illogical in their sequence. Circumstantiality is a disorder of association by which too little selective suppression of ideas allows too many associated concepts to come into consciousness. The connection between ideas, however, is usually logical and easy to follow.

Difficulty holding on to a train of thought—blocking—often manifests as an interruption in the middle of a thought. The sentence following such an interruption may have no relationship to what has just been said. Blocking, which is thought to be due to an intensification of anxiety, is not a conscious mechanism and thus not subject to conscious control.

Magical thinking is displayed by children, people affected by a variety of psychiatric conditions, and some primitive peoples. Essentially, it is a belief that specific thoughts, words, or gestures can directly lead to the fulfillment of wishes. Such thinking demonstrates an unrealistic understanding of the relationship between cause and effect.

Depersonalization is the sense of being outside one's own body, observing oneself as an actor engaged in a role. This symptom may be manifested by people suffering from temporary anxiety, neurotic (especially phobic) people, and severely mentally ill people, such as certain schizophrenics. Some people with an organic brain disorder, such as temporal lobe epilepsy, may develop both depersonalization and derealization, the feeling that one's surroundings are unfamiliar or unreal.

45-47. The answers are: 45-B, 46-A, 47-D. *(Talbott, pp 72-74.)* When using assessment instruments, the clinician or researcher must be assured the test is valid and reliable. Validity refers to the test's ability to assess what it claims to be assessing. Reliability refers to the reproducibility of results at various times. An unreliable test will not produce consistent results. Statistical significance refers to the results and how often they would happen by chance. A p value of less than 0.05 is statistically significant and means the results would only happen 5 times out of 100 by chance.

Human Behavior: Theories of Personality and Development

DIRECTIONS: Each question below contains five suggested responses. Select the one best response to each question.

48. The large majority of mentally retarded persons are mildly retarded, with IQs on standard psychological tests of

(A) below 20
(B) 20 to 34
(C) 35 to 49
(D) 50 to 70
(E) 71 to 85

49. Sexual drive, when defined as the spontaneous manifestation of genital excitement, is believed by most clinicians to

(A) peak at an earlier age in women
(B) be generally strongest during young adulthood
(C) be virtually nonexistent after the age of 60
(D) be reduced by elevated prolactin
(E) be androgen-dependent only in the male

50. Modern psychoanalytic theory holds that narcissism is

(A) a pathologic state
(B) a normal part of human personality development
(C) the most frequent cause of hypersexuality
(D) first manifested during the oedipal period
(E) of little consequence except in children

51. Which of the following theorists primarily focused on the maturation of the sense of self from infantile fragility and fragmentation into the cohesive and stable structure of adulthood?

(A) Piaget
(B) Erikson
(C) Freud
(D) Klein
(E) Kohut

52. Tourette's disorder is characterized by

(A) onset between ages 15 and 30
(B) sleep disturbance
(C) sexual dysfunction
(D) multiple motor and vocal tics
(E) episodes of panic

53. All the following statements about the psychoanalytic concept of the oedipal phase of development are true EXCEPT that

(A) it occurs between the phallic and the latency stages
(B) it is usually followed by identification with the parent of the same sex
(C) it occurs only in the development of children destined to become neurotic
(D) it is associated with the phenomenon of castration anxiety
(E) it occurs in both males and females

54. While homosexuality remains a controversial subject within psychiatry, most contemporary psychiatrists consider it to be a

(A) personality disorder
(B) neurosis
(C) genetically based brain disorder
(D) form of pathologic sexuality
(E) variant of sexual preference

55. Identity diffusion, as described by Erik Erikson, occurs primarily during

(A) infancy
(B) childhood
(C) adolescence
(D) adulthood
(E) old age

56. The early studies of Réné Spitz suggested that

(A) disturbed mothers are instrumental in causing behavioral problems in early infancy
(B) infants reared with little maternal contact are more susceptible to infections and behavioral problems
(C) infants reared in an institutional setting are likely to become autistic
(D) the number of toys available to infants is a crucial factor in their development
(E) environmental variables have little impact on the health of infants

57. All the following statements concerning children's IQ scores are true EXCEPT that

(A) the scores can vary widely if an individual child is tested more than once
(B) the scores can increase over time in children who are highly motivated
(C) the scores correlate fairly well with achievement in school
(D) the scores are determined predominantly by heredity
(E) the mean of the scores remains fairly constant within a given group

58. Piaget is best known for his theories and investigations of

(A) cognitive development
(B) affective component of development
(C) mood-related development
(D) motor development
(E) kinesthetic development

59. Children diagnosed as having
attention-deficit disorder, also called
minimal brain dysfunction (MBD),
would be LEAST likely to display
which of the following signs?

(A) Impulsivity
(B) Hyperactivity
(C) Emotional lability
(D) Severe neurologic deficits
(E) Perceptual motor impairments

DIRECTIONS: Each question below contains four suggested responses of which one or more is correct. Select

A	if	1, 2, and 3	are correct
B	if	1 and 3	are correct
C	if	2 and 4	are correct
D	if	4	is correct
E	if	1, 2, 3, and 4	are correct

60. True statements about REM sleep include which of the following?

(1) The proportion and duration of REM sleep decrease from birth to adulthood

(2) Most adults spend 80 to 100 minutes each night in REM sleep, which is associated with three to six separate dreams

(3) REM sleep is not the only state in which dreams can occur

(4) Depressed patients who are deprived of REM sleep have a marked worsening of their condition

61. True statements about the human immune system include

(1) exposure to psychosocial stress can alter a variety of components of immune function

(2) it is highly unlikely that early life experiences will alter the immune system in later life

(3) immune response has been found to be subject to conditioning effects

(4) immune abnormalities have been shown to be involved in the pathogenesis of schizophrenia

62. Patients with Down's syndrome often display

(1) chromosomal abnormalities

(2) hypotonia and hyperflexibility

(3) a flat nasal bridge

(4) shortness of ear length

63. True statements about sleepwalking include

(1) 15 percent of children from the ages of 5 to 12 sleepwalk at least once

(2) sleepwalking in children is usually not associated with psychopathology

(3) sleepwalking is potentially dangerous and requires precautions to protect the child

(4) a psychological cause is suggested when sleepwalking begins in adolescence or adulthood

64. In psychoanalytic theory, the superego

(1) contains the ego ideal, an internalized set of standards

(2) contains the unconscious conscience

(3) demands punishment in the form of guilt and shame

(4) is the source of the psychological defense mechanisms that repress unacceptable impulses

65. Children with attention-deficit disorder

(1) often fidget and are restless
(2) persevere in a single activity
(3) often talk excessively
(4) are obsessively careful to avoid dangerous play

66. True statements about the expressive movements of the human face in infancy include

(1) smiling and expressions of disgust appear at birth
(2) by 9 months of age infants can produce most adult emotional expressions
(3) babies who are blind at birth display expressions of anger, fear, sadness, and happiness
(4) by the age of 2 months, infants are using facial expression to communicate with adults

67. True statements regarding the differences between men and women include which of the following?

(1) Women have a higher prevalence rate of affective disorders
(2) Men have a higher prevalence rate of anxiety disorders
(3) Prevalence rates of personality disorders are consistently higher for men
(4) Women have a prevalence rate of schizophrenia that is twice that for men

68. Psychoanalytic theory describes the ego as a coherent system of functions, including

(1) regulation of instinctual drives
(2) defense formation
(3) formation of relationships
(4) adaptation to reality

69. Freud's theory of infantile sexual development can be described by which of the following statements?

(1) It postulates that sexuality begins in early infancy
(2) It links neurosis with disturbance in psychosexual development
(3) It describes the earliest sexuality as centered in the mouth, lips, and tongue
(4) It suggests that masturbation normally begins during the latency period

70. Childhood stuttering is accurately described by which of the following statements?

(1) Affected children usually have obsessive compulsive personality traits
(2) Affected children often outgrow the problem
(3) Girls are affected more commonly than boys
(4) A family history of stuttering frequently is elicited

SUMMARY OF DIRECTIONS

A	B	C	D	E
1, 2, 3	1, 3	2, 4	4	All are
only	only	only	only	correct

71. According to classic psycho-analytic theory, correct statements about the phallic phase of development include which of the following?

(1) It marks the start of the oedipal conflict
(2) It occurs after 5 years of age
(3) It is characterized by sexual curiosity and comparison
(4) It does not occur in girls

72. Primary process thinking is a psychoanalytic concept describing mental activity that is

(1) typically unconscious
(2) prelogical and primitive
(3) manifested in dreams
(4) prominent in psychosis

73. Harry Stack Sullivan's theory of personality development is characterized by which of the following concepts?

(1) An emphasis on the importance of interpersonal relations
(2) A conviction that the basic structure of personality is fixed by about 5 years of age
(3) A concern with the developmental impact of social position and life style
(4) A focus on ego psychology

74. Current evidence suggests that genetic (inherited) factors may play an important role in which of the following disorders?

(1) Bipolar disorder
(2) Tourette's syndrome
(3) Schizophrenia
(4) Alzheimer's disease

75. The developmental theories of Erikson and Freud differ in that

(1) Erikson minimizes the role of the unconscious, while Freud emphasizes it
(2) Erikson emphasizes the interplay of cultural factors with individual psychological development to a greater degree than Freud
(3) Erikson's is a behavioral theory, while Freud's is an analytic theory
(4) Erikson places greater emphasis than Freud on ego structures

76. Correct statements concerning infantile autism include which of the following?

(1) It may occur during the first few months of life
(2) It usually is not associated with language disturbances
(3) It may manifest itself in resistance to minor environmental changes
(4) Affected infants form abnormally intense attachments to adults

77. Correct statements about adopted children include which of the following?

(1) They should be told of their adoption between ages 7 and 10, according to many experts
(2) They usually search for their biologic parents only if their adoptive family relations are seriously troubled
(3) They are more likely to display behavioral problems, learning difficulties, and minimal brain dysfunction than are nonadopted children
(4) They often are painfully disillusioned if they succeed in finding and meeting their biologic parents

78. Battered or abused children are

(1) abused most commonly by their fathers
(2) usually from very poor families
(3) most frequently between 3 and 6 years of age when the diagnosis is made
(4) typically born to parents who were abused when they were children

79. Correct statements concerning the latency stage of development include which of the following?

(1) It follows resolution of the Oedipus complex
(2) It consolidates identification with the parent of the same sex
(3) It involves wider peer contact
(4) It is the phase of identity crisis

80. In psychoanalytic theory, the anal phase of development, which occurs between the ages of approximately 1 and 3 years, is characterized by

(1) struggles over routines
(2) depressive episodes
(3) striving for independence
(4) head banging

DIRECTIONS: Each group of questions below consists of lettered headings followed by a set of numbered items. For each numbered item select the **one** lettered heading with which it is **most** closely associated. Each lettered heading may be used once, **more than once**, or **not at all**.

Questions 81–83

The concept of defenses is central to psychoanalytic theory. Match each of the definitions below to the defense mechanism being described.

(A) Acting out
(B) Rationalization
(C) Isolation
(D) Repression
(E) Sublimation

81. The unconscious exclusion of an idea or feeling from conscious awareness

82. The intrapsychic separation of affect and mental content

83. The direct behavioral expression of an unconscious impulse

---

Questions 84–87

Match the following.

(A) Core-gender identity
(B) Gender-role behavior
(C) Gender-role identity
(D) Sexual identity
(E) Sex print

84. The internal experience of sexual arousal patterns and self-labeling

85. The inner conviction that one is a male or one is a female

86. The person's self-evaluation of psychological maleness or femaleness

87. The objective patterns of sexuality

Questions 88–91

For each age below, select the psychosocial crisis, as described by Erikson, with which it is most likely to be associated.

(A) Identity versus role confusion
(B) Generativity versus stagnation
(C) Integrity versus despair
(D) Initiative versus guilt
(E) Industry versus inferiority

88. 5 years of age

89. 15 years of age

90. 40 years of age

91. 65 years of age

Questions 92-95

Match the following.

(A) Neutralization
(B) Wish fulfillment
(C) Identification
(D) Secondary gain
(E) Overdetermination

92. The concept that a symptom may have a number of different origins and meanings

93. The process by which libidinal and aggressive drives are mastered and provide conflict-free energy

94. The benefit derived as a result of neurotic illness

95. The unconscious process by which persons pattern themselves after others

Questions 96-99

For each psychic phenomenon or experience listed below, select the psychoanalytic theorist with whom it is most commonly associated.

(A) Sigmund Freud
(B) Harry Stack Sullivan
(C) John Bowlby
(D) Melanie Klein
(E) Carl Jung
(F) Heinz Kohut
(G) Erich Fromm

96. Signal anxiety as a result of conflict between the id, ego, and superego

97. Relationship problems determined by the occurrence of empathic failures and developmental arrests

98. Anxiety highly determined by developmental bonding and attachment behavior

99. Personality styles influenced by archetypal modes of experience

Human Behavior:
Theories of Personality
and Development

Answers

48. The answer is D. *(American Psychiatric Association, ed 3-R, pp 28–33.)* Mild retardation refers to the condition of those persons whose IQ tests are between 50 and 70 on standard tests such as the Stanford-Binet or Wechsler. These people constitute about 85 percent of those with mental retardation and are often not distinguishable from other children until later in childhood. They can be expected to learn academic skills up to approximately the sixth-grade level, and with proper social and vocational education they can achieve minimum levels of self-support as adults.

49. The answer is D. *(American Psychiatric Association, Treatments, pp 2265–2266.)* Sexual desire can be clinically best understood as a composite of sexual drive, motivation, and aspiration. Sexual drive is an androgen-dependent system in both males and females. It has a frequency that varies over the life cycle and is generally strongest in adolescence. Many persons over the age of 60 continue to experience sexual drive, though reduced compared with earlier developmental phases. Most clinicians believe that sexual drive declines after the twenties in males and after the thirties for most females. Elevated prolactin levels from pituitary tumors or phenothiazines are associated with decreased sexual drive.

50. The answer is B. *(Nemiroff, pp 73–81.)* Narcissism, or self-love, is a major concept in modern psychoanalytic theory. It is viewed as a normal part of the development of all children, beginning in infancy. It can become a pathologic issue in the presence of developmental conflict or deficit. Although it ultimately may become linked to sexuality, in and of itself it does not imply genital sexuality. It may be a contributing factor in hypersexuality, but certainly is not the major cause in most cases. Narcissism is an important contributing factor in self-esteem and is of significance throughout the life cycle.

51. The answer is E. *(Kaplan, ed 5. pp 366–367, 1443–1445. Michels, vol 1, chap 1, pp 2–15.)* Heinz Kohut developed a variant of psychoanalysis that has had a powerful influence on modern psychoanalytic treatment. He believed that psychic development was primarily organized around the developmental vicissitudes of the self, especially in the relationship to interactions with self-objects. The most important self-object of infancy is the mother. Freudian psychoanalysis postulated a sequence of psychosexual development that stressed unconscious conflict and the influence of sexual and aggressive drives. Erik Erikson elaborated the role of culture in shaping the meaning of these drives throughout the life cycle. Melanie Klein is associated with the object-relations school of psychoanalysis, especially a minute dissection of the early relationship of the child and mother. Piaget is particularly known for his work on the development of intellect.

52.   The answer is D. (*American Psychiatric Association, ed 3-R, pp 79-80.*) Tourette's disorder has its onset before age 21 and is characterized by multiple motor and vocal tics that have been present during the illness, although not necessarily concurrently. A tic is defined as an involuntary, sudden, rapid, recurrent, nonrhythmic, and stereotyped motor movement or vocalization. It is experienced as irresistible and exacerbated by stress. Sometimes it can be suppressed. Tics are usually diminished during sleep.

53.   The answer is C. (*Kaplan, ed 5. pp 364-365.*) According to psychoanalytic theory, the oedipal phase of development occurs in all male and female children. It occurs during the third to fifth years, that is, between the phallic and latency periods. It is related to the Oedipus complex—namely, sexual striving toward the parent of the opposite sex and jealous and murderous fantasies toward the parent of the same sex. Oedipal striving is normally abandoned in the male because of castration anxiety, and in the female because of mother's disapproval and father's failure to comply. In both cases, this leads to a period of more intense identification with the parent of the same sex.

54.   The answer is E. (*Talbott, pp 600-601.*) While homosexuality was formerly considered to be a sexual disorder, the current view of the American Psychiatric Association is that homosexuality should not be considered a mental disorder but rather a variant of sexual preference. This change was in part based on accumulated evidence that the rate and type of psychopathology is no different in homosexuals than in heterosexuals. The etiology of homosexuality remains obscure and controversial. Many psychiatrists believe there is a biologic vulnerability, which is then acted upon by psychological issues in the course of development.

55.   The answer is C. (*Kaplan, ed 5. pp 115, 119.*) Erikson discussed at length the turbulence of adolescence, and the fact that it was a period of development wherein the individual was deeply involved in solidifying a sense of identity. Identity for Erikson included a continuity with one's past, a sense of sameness as well as a solid sense of self that includes goals, aims, and life style, as well as sexual identity. Identity diffusion, which occurs to some degree in all adolescents and most markedly in troubled adolescents, is characterized by confusion, insecurity, and aimlessness.

56. The answer is B. *(Nicholi, p 609.)* René A. Spitz's pioneering studies on the effects of institutionalization on infants compared three groups of children: those reared by their delinquent mothers in the nursery of a penal institution; those reared in a foundling home with no maternal contact; and those reared in two-parent home environments. The infants raised in the foundling home showed a markedly higher incidence of disease and developmental delay. The key factor that differentiated this group from the others was the lack of maternal contact and not the type of mothering, institutional setting, or play environment.

57. The answer is D. *(Kaplan, ed 5. pp 497–499.)* IQ scores, which correlate fairly well with school achievement, can vary widely in an individual child tested more than once. In one study, the scores of more than two-thirds of the tested children varied by more than 15 points over a specified period of time. Despite such individual variation, however, the mean IQ of a given group remains quite constant. Children who at 5 years of age display high levels of independence and self-initiative are more likely to show subsequent IQ gains. There have not been any adequate studies demonstrating that IQ is determined predominantly by heredity.

58. The answer is A. *(Kaplan, ed 5. pp 98–101.)* Piaget was a pioneer in the investigation of intelligent behavior. His interest was primarily in the cognitive development of children, and the affective component of development was of lesser interest to him. He elaborated stages of cognitive development from the sensory motor intelligence of infants to the abstract operations and thinking that become important in early adolescence.

59. The answer is D. *(Kaplan, ed 5. pp 1829–1834.)* Attention-deficit disorder is characterized by hyperactivity, distractibility, emotional lability, perceptual motor defects, learning problems, and short attention span. Neurologic examination of affected children may reveal no abnormalities or may show minimal, nonspecific signs, including hearing and speech deficits and coordination problems. Electro-encephalography often reveals a variety of nonspecific abnormalities, though testing in a significant percentage of affected children provides normal results.

60. The answer is A (1, 2, 3). *(Michels, vol 3, chap 60, pp 2–10.)* Sleep is usually classified into rapid and nonrapid eye movement (REM and NREM) sleep. Most adults have three to six dreams per night during an average of 1 to 2 h of REM sleep. Dreaming is particularly associated with REM sleep, but it can also occur during NREM sleep, when it has a tendency to be more conceptual than perceptual. The normal newborn's REM sleep is about 50 percent of total sleep, but by 2 to 3 years of age the child reaches the adult level of 20 to 25 percent. Depriving depressed patients of REM sleep appears to have an antidepressant effect.

61.   The answer is B (1, 3). *(Michels, vol 2, chap 128, pp 1-14.)* The effects of stress on the immune system, as well as responsiveness to conditioning, are well established in animals. Evidence is similarly accumulating regarding humans. A number of investigators have demonstrated that early life experience may alter the immune system so that the effects persist into later life. Research has failed to yet establish a relationship between pathology in the immune system and schizophrenia. However, it is clear that the immune system is modulated by psychosocial events via effects on the central nervous system and endocrine processes.

62.   The answer is E (all). *(Kaplan, ed 5. pp 1739-1741.)* The diagnosis of Down's syndrome is ultimately made by study of the chromosomes. While there is no physical anomaly invariably present, the vast majority of patients display hypotonia, hyperflexibility, midface depression, and short ear length. Other common physical findings include oblique palpebral fissures, loose skin on the back of the neck, and gaps between the first and second toes.

63.   The answer is E (all). *(Michels, vol 2, chap 43, pp 6-8; vol 2, chap 52, p 6.)* While 15 percent of children will sleepwalk at least once, in only a much smaller percentage does it become recurrent and persistent. Usually the problem will resolve spontaneously by the age of 15, though sometimes it becomes associated with the problem of night terrors. Studies of adult somnambulists have found a large percentage with demonstrable psychiatric problems. It is quite possible for a child to be injured while sleepwalking, since it is not purposeful behavior. It has been postulated that sleepwalking and night terrors share a common physiologic origin for which there may be a genetic predisposition.

64.   The answer is A (1, 2, 3). *(Michels, vol 1, chap 1, p 9.)* The superego is the "site" of the ego ideal and of the conscience. It sits in judgment as to whether one's behavior and wishes are right, wrong, good, bad, or shameful. It is a largely unconscious process and does not distinguish between thoughts and acts. For this reason, it produces guilt about wish and fantasy, not merely about the person's deeds.

65.   The answer is B (1, 3). *(American Psychiatric Association, ed 3-R. pp 50-53.)* Attention-deficit disorder has its onset before age 7 and is a disturbance of at least 6 months' duration. The symptoms include hyperactivity, impulsive speech and behavior, and easy distractibility. Patients often have difficulty in maintaining attention on one activity and in listening to others. An important management problem relates to the tendency to engage in dangerous behavior without considering the consequences.

66.   The answer is E (all). *(Kaplan, ed 5. pp 1695-1708.)* There is an extensive literature on the facial expressions of infants, and the preponderance of evidence suggests that this activity is innate. Even blind babies will smile while fixating toward their mother's voice, in addition to showing other emotional expressiveness.

While visual learning provides an important element in the development of normal expressive behavior, innate factors are clearly operative.

67.   The answer is B (1, 3). *(Kaplan, ed 5. pp 302, 322–325.)* The differences between males and females as to prevalence of mental and emotional disorders reflect a complex interaction between biologic and sociocultural factors. The sexes are treated differently with respect to expectations, social roles, social opportunities, and so forth. All these factors operate throughout the life cycle to shape behavior and responses to the environment. Women have been shown to have a greater prevalence rate of affective disorders and anxiety disorders, and a lesser rate of personality disorders. There are slight and perhaps not significantly different rates for schizophrenia and organic brain syndromes associated with aging.

68.   The answer is E (all). *(Kaplan, ed 5. pp 372–374.)* The ego mediates between a person's instincts and the outside world. It is the part of the personality that perceives stimuli and can respond to them through control of both the id and voluntary muscular responses. Its many functions include reality testing, the formation and regulation of defenses, and the establishment of relationships with others.

69.   The answer is A (1, 2, 3). *(Kaplan, ed 5. pp 362–364.)* Freud postulated the existence of three phases of infantile psychosexual development. The oral phase lasts for the first year to year and a half of life, a time during which an infant's needs, perceptions, and pleasures are centered in the mouth, lips, and tongue. Masturbation begins in early infancy and peaks in the phallic phase and again at puberty. Psychoanalytic theory links neurosis with disturbances in psychosexual development—Freud observed that many of his patients had distorted memories of early sexual experiences, confusing infantile sexual fantasy with actual events.

70.   The answer is C (2, 4). *(Kaplan, ed 5. pp 1810–1811.)* The causes of stuttering are not known. Although the incidence of stuttering in the relatives of stutterers is higher than in the general population, the genetic contribution to the development of stuttering is unclear. Stuttering affects boys more often and more chronically than girls. Treatment is controversial; however, 40 percent or more of affected young children eventually outgrow the difficulty. No particular personality classification is typical of persons who stutter.

71.   The answer is B (1, 3). *(Kaplan, ed 5. pp 362, 364.)* According to classic psychoanalytic theory, the phallic phase of development begins at approximately 3 years of age and lasts about 2 years. During this time the erotic preoccupations of both boys and girls shift from the anal to the genital areas of the body. Children in this phase become sexually curious, comparing themselves with each other and with their parents. They compete for the attention of the parent of the opposite sex and are buffeted by intense and conflict-laden relations with both parents. This phenomenon, the Oedipus complex, plays a critical role in the pathogenesis of neurotic disorders.

72.   The answer is E (all). *(Kaplan, ed 5. pp 560–561.)* Psychoanalytic theory describes primary process thinking as mental activity related to the id. It is pre-logical, timeless, primitive, and associated with the tendency to seek immediate gratification. It is characteristic of infancy, dreams, and psychotic thinking, but it is largely unconscious in normal waking life. Secondary process thinking is related to the activity of the ego. It is organized, logical, responsive to the demands of reality, and, unlike primary process thinking, usually conscious.

73.   The answer is B (1, 3). *(Kaplan, ed 5. pp 424–427.)* Harry Stack Sullivan is best known for his theory of personality development, which emphasizes the central importance of interpersonal relations. Sullivan believed that the first 5 years of life, though crucial to psychological development, do not fully fix personality; instead, personality continues to develop and change throughout adolescence and even into adulthood. He emphasized the influence of social position and conditions on development. Sullivan's theory focuses on a complex concept of the self, which differs in important respects from the psychoanalytic concept of the ego.

74.   The answer is E (all). *(Kaplan, ed 5. pp 4, 614, 732–744, 879–880.)* Although conclusive proof is lacking, studies of twins, adopted children, and biochemical data suggest that many psychiatric disorders have a significant genetic component. The data are particularly strong for affective disorders. Current evidence indicates there are at least three genetic forms of bipolar disorder. Data from family histories and from biochemical studies suggest that Tourette's syndrome has an inherited basis. Schizophrenia remains more controversial, but a reasonable interpretation of the evidence indicates that both inherited *and* environmental factors contribute to the disorder. Although a clear-cut pattern of genetic predisposition to Alzheimer's disease has not emerged, well-documented familial cases exist, some of which follow an autosomal dominant pattern of inheritance.

75.   The answer is C (2, 4). *(Colarusso, pp 27–33. Kaplan, ed 5. pp 403–409.)* The developmental theories of both Freud and Erikson are psychoanalytic and acknowledge the role of the unconscious. Erikson, however, is more concerned with the individual's development as it relates to the surrounding cultural milieu. Consistent with more recent psychoanalytic theory, Erikson also emphasizes ego psychology in his formulations.

76.   The answer is B (1, 3). *(Kaplan, ed 5. pp 1778–1780.)* Infantile autism manifests itself quite early in life and is often associated with a language disturbance. Children with infantile autism have an extreme desire to avoid all change. These children tend to lack any interest in forming normal attachments to other people.

77. The answer is B (1, 3). *(Kaplan, ed 5. pp 1958-1961.)* The consensus among adoption experts is that adopted children should be told of their adoption sometime between 7 and 10 years of age. Adopted children appear to develop behavioral problems and learning difficulties more often than other children. Moreover, adopted children born to teenage mothers may have an increased incidence of a variety of neurologic disorders, perhaps because of poor prenatal and obstetric care. Mature adoptees usually are interested in their biologic parents (birth parents) and may search for them. Most adoptees find reunion with their birth parents a positive experience that often leads them to form a closer relationship with their adoptive parents.

78. The answer is D (4). *(Kaplan, ed 5. 1962-1968.)* Although child abuse can affect children of any age, children less than 3 years of age are affected most frequently and most severely. Mothers, more often than fathers, are the abusers. Abusing parents commonly were abused when they were children, and families in which child abuse occurs can be found in all socioeconomic strata.

79. The answer is A (1, 2, 3). *(Kaplan, ed 5. pp 377-378.)* The latency stage of development follows the resolution of the Oedipus complex and lasts until adolescence (i.e., from approximately 5 to 13 years of age). During this period, children consolidate their sense of identification with parents of the same sex and develop an active fantasy life. Cognitive skills are expanded, and contacts with significant, extrafamilial figures (e.g., in school) widen. Identity crisis is a term coined by Erikson to describe another stage of development—adolescence.

80. The answer is B (1, 3). *(Kaplan, ed 5. p 364.)* In the anal phase of development, children struggle with their parents over eating, toilet training, sleeping, and other situations in which their autonomy is brought into question. Whether depressive-type episodes occur during the anal period is controversial; the clinicians who believe that these episodes do occur consider their presence highly pathologic. Because head banging occurs more frequently earlier in life, its occurrence during the anal phase should suggest the need for psychiatric evaluation.

81-83. The answers are: 81-D, 82-C, 83-A. *(Kaplan, ed 5. pp 374-376.)* Psychoanalytic theory postulates that every person, normal or neurotic, uses defenses. Some defenses, such as altruism (vicarious gratification by service to others) and sublimation (gratification of a potentially objectionable impulse by socially acceptable means), are considered to be mature and healthy. Repression, isolation, and rationalization are neurotic defenses. Repression, which plays a primary role in the pathogenesis of hysteria, involves the unconscious exclusion of a thought or feeling from conscious awareness. It is often associated with symbolic behavior representing expression of the repressed mental content. Isolation involves separating painful feelings from the thoughts provoking them. Both the thoughts and attendant affect may be excluded from awareness or the affect may be displaced onto a different thought altogether. Rationalization involves supporting unacceptable ideas or behavior by basically inaccurate but plausible explanations. Acting out is an immature defense in which an inner conflict can be partially and transiently relieved by unconscious expression in impulsive action.

84-87. The answers are: 84-D, 85-A, 86-C, 87-E. *(Michels, vol 1, chap 46, pp 1-2.)* Sexual identity refers to how a person subjectively experiences his or her sexual arousal patterns. It includes an awareness of what is experienced as erotic and desirable and is a part of one's overall sense of self. For example, a person who experiences both homosexual and heterosexual erotic arousal might consult a psychiatrist because of confusion about sexual identity.

Core-gender identity reflects a self-image of one's biologic sex. It therefore represents the person's self-designation as being female or male. Generally it corresponds to biologic sex, but it may be ambiguous in certain hermaphroditic conditions as well as in gender identity disorders such as transsexualism.

Gender-role identity refers to a person's self-image and self-evaluation that results in a belief that "I am male" or "I am female." It develops well into adulthood and fluctuates sometimes as a reflection of the person's evaluation of feelings, behavior, and performance. It is closely connected to the degree to which one feels one has adequately met the prescribed cultural role.

The sex print refers to objective patterns of sexuality. It is more comprehensive than preference for a particular sexual object or a specific sexual activity, but is the deep-rooted script that is most able to elicit erotic desire. It contributes to the person's sexual identity (subjective self-labeling), but forms the objective patterns that determine the substance of the person's sexual fantasies and behavior.

88-91. The answers are: 88-D, 89-A, 90-B, 91-C. *(Colarusso, pp 27-33, Kaplan, ed 5. pp 405-409.)* Erikson described the personality development of humans in terms of eight major, sequential stages. While acknowledging Freud's psychosexual developmental theory, Erikson broadened the scope of his formulations by including social factors outside the parent-child triad, by shifting the emphasis from psychopathologic constructs to issues of normal growth and development, and by concluding that the process of development is a lifelong one. The resolution of each of the eight stages of development depends, Erikson said, on mastery of prior stages and influences the course of subsequent stages.

In the oral-sensory stage (the first year of life), trust versus mistrust is the important issue. In the second stage, corresponding to the Freudian anal period, successful resolution results in autonomy; problems in this stage can result in shame or self-doubt. The third stage lasts through the fifth year of life and parallels the Freudian period characterized by the emergence of the Oedipus complex. Erikson describes the task of this stage as the healthy growth initiative. During latency, years 6 to 11, industry versus inferiority is the important psychosocial crisis. Building on the autonomy and initiative of earlier stages, children approach the tasks of adult life. Whether industry flourishes or feelings of inferiority arise depends on children's interactions with teachers and peers, as well as with parents. Erikson's ideas about the development of identity during adolescence are particularly well known. He felt that, during this period, adolescents try to integrate and clarify their own identities in relation to their parents, peers, and members of the opposite sex; if they are unsuccessful, role confusion can result.

Although Freud believed that the reworking of the Oedipus complex in adolescence was the final stage of development, Erikson saw development continuing into adulthood. He saw intimacy versus isolation to be the primary crisis of young adults. During the years of middle age, generativity versus stagnation is the key issue. Erikson emphasized the importance not only of rearing children but also of engaging in activities to help others, particularly new generations. In the final stage, people reflect on their lives. Adequate resolution of the stages of intimacy and generativity provides contentment in this stage (integrity); poor resolution can foster despair and a debilitating fear of death.

92-95. The answers are: 92-E, 93-A, 94-D, 95-C. *(Kaplan, ed 5. pp 372, 1014, 1444-1445, 1451-1452.)* Each of the terms listed in the question describes a concept important to psychoanalytic theory. Neutralization is the term suggested by Heinz Hartmann to describe the process by which libidinal and aggressive drives are mastered, thus freeing energy for the ego. This concept is important in helping to explain nondefensive ego functioning. Overdetermination describes the concept that mental phenomena, such as neurotic symptoms and dreams, have multiple causes and thus have multiple meanings.

Identification is a defense that plays an important role in normal development. It involves unconscious patterning after another person, producing structural change in the ego.

Primary gain refers to the relief of tension and conflict produced by the development of neurotic symptoms. In addition to the internal reduction of distress, neurotic persons may attempt to derive compensation or gratification from the external world (secondary gain) as a result of their suffering. Examples of secondary gain include an increase in attention and sympathy, relief from burdensome obligations, and monetary compensation.

Wish fulfillment is the term used by Freud to describe the primary goal of dreams.

96-99. The answers are: 96-A, 97-F, 98-C, 99-E. *(Kaplan, ed 5. pp 132-135, 142, 144-145, 153-154.)* In the structural theory, Freud proposed three divisions of the mind: id, ego, and superego. This was an advance over the topographical theory, which elaborated the concepts of the conscious and unconscious. The id is the site of the pleasure-oriented drives; the ego is the central mediating agency charged with interfacing with the id, the superego (conscience and ideals), and reality. Conflict, generating signal anxiety, occurs when unacceptable id impulses threaten to become conscious or to result in behavior unacceptable to the superego a l ego.

Heinz Kohut was originally a classical psychoanalyst who later developed a system of psychoanalysis that is most often referred to as self-psychology. Rather than focusing on instincts and conflict, Kohut stressed the development of the self, particularly as it relates to developmental deficits and failures in phase-appropriate empathy. The development of a cohesive sense of self and self-esteem is seen as the most critical developmental task.

John Bowlby is usually classified among the psychoanalytic developmentalists. His studies suggest a primary bonding drive with age-related phases particularly important during infancy. This is expressed in attachment behavior consisting of clinging, sucking, following, crying, and smiling. He made the parent-child relationship central and not subservient to drive discharge.

Carl Jung was originally a member of Freud's inner circle, but later split with him largely over questions of libido, psychic energy, and the nature of the unconscious. Jung believed the unconscious was more than the product of personal history, but also included a collective unconscious with memories of our cultural past, racial memory, and even prehuman memory. The unconscious contains archetypes, which are innate ideas that have accumulated over generations and then interact with life experiences. Archetypes include innate ideas about such things as mother, father, hero, and the masculine and feminine prototypes within us.

Human Behavior: Biologic and Related Sciences

DIRECTIONS: Each question below contains five suggested responses. Select the **one best** response to each question.

100. Synaptic communication in the brain is accomplished via which of the following mechanisms?

(A) Chemical only
(B) Electrical only
(C) A combination of chemical and electrical events
(D) Mechanical only
(E) None of the above

101. The highest density of cholinergic innervation of any brain structure is found in the

(A) cerebral cortex
(B) caudate nucleus and putamen
(C) cerebellum
(D) spinal cord
(E) locus ceruleus

102. Hypothalamic function is closely related to all the following EXCEPT

(A) sleep
(B) appetite
(C) memory
(D) sexual behavior
(E) fear

103. Biologic rhythms—cyclic, internally regulated bodily responses—are operative in all the following EXCEPT

(A) birth rate
(B) death
(C) body temperature
(D) personality disorders
(E) depression

104. Deprivation of REM sleep is associated with which of the following?

(A) Onset of psychosis
(B) Dementia-like syndrome
(C) Improvement in depression
(D) Development of personality disorders
(E) Onset of acute anxiety

105. The highest prevalence of tardive dyskinesia has been observed in

(A) elderly females
(B) young females
(C) elderly males
(D) young males
(E) male and female infants

106. Most studies suggest that the major inhibitory neurotransmitter in the brain is

(A) serotonin
(B) dopamine
(C) beta-endorphin
(D) γ-aminobutyric acid
(E) somatostatin

107. True statements concerning cataplexy include which of the following?

(A) Cataplexy is associated with unconsciousness
(B) Cataplexy involves sudden loss of muscle tone
(C) Cataplexy is unrelated to emotional states
(D) Cataplexy can last up to an hour
(E) Cataplexy is best treated with neuroleptics

108. Typical behavior in patients displaying the catastrophic reaction, as defined by Goldstein (1939) and Gainotti (1972), include all the following EXCEPT

(A) restlessness and hypermotility
(B) ingratiating behavior toward the examiner
(C) sudden bursts of tears
(D) cursing
(E) refusal to continue the examination

109. The dietary amino-acid precursor of catecholamines is

(A) tryptophan
(B) glutamic acid
(C) aspartic acid
(D) tyrosine
(E) glycine

110. In the absence of other symptoms, sporadically occurring behavioral automatisms and olfactory hallucinations suggest the diagnosis of

(A) schizophrenia
(B) schizophreniform psychosis
(C) hysterical personality disorder
(D) nondominant parietal lobe lesion
(E) temporal lobe lesion

111. For a substance to be classified as a neurotransmitter, all the following must be true EXCEPT

(A) the substance must be concentrated in the presynaptic nerve terminal
(B) the substance must be released by a depolarizing stimulus applied to the neuron
(C) the effects on the postsynaptic receptor are the same whether the substance is released from the presynaptic neuron or applied exogenously
(D) the neuron must be able to synthesize the substance
(E) there must be no mechanism for inactivation of the substance after its release from the presynaptic nerve terminal

112. Which of the following types of studies offers the most promise in elucidating the interaction between genetic and environmental factors in psychiatric illness?

(A) Family risk studies
(B) Twin studies
(C) Adoption studies
(D) Genetic marker studies
(E) Prospective longitudinal studies

113. Information is transmitted along a neuron in a series of electrochemical events known as

(A) translators
(B) resting potentials
(C) polarity maintainers
(D) action potentials
(E) none of the above

114. The group of neurotransmitters known as biogenic amines include all the following EXCEPT

(A) γ-aminobutyric acid (GABA)
(B) serotonin
(C) dopamine
(D) acetylcholine
(E) epinephrine

DIRECTIONS: Each question below contains four suggested responses of which **one or more** is correct. Select

A	if	**1, 2, and 3**	are correct
B	if	1 and 3	are correct
C	if	**2 and 4**	are correct
D	if	4	is correct
E	if	**1, 2, 3, and 4**	are correct

115. Studies used to determine the genetic influence in emotional disorders include

(1) twin studies

(2) studies of adoptees and their families

(3) studies of familial risk

(4) studies of drug responses in family members

116. During the last month, a 42-year-old woman who is recently widowed has displayed a markedly dysphoric mood, has lost 6.8 kg (15 lb), has been extremely lethargic, and has experienced vaguely suicidal thoughts. She is in good physical health and has had no previous psychiatric contact. The type of medication most likely to be chosen for the treatment of this woman is thought to act by

(1) increasing postsynaptic receptor sensitivity to serotonin

(2) decreasing plasma levels of dopamine-β-hydroxylase

(3) blocking norepinephrine uptake into synaptic terminals

(4) blocking the accumulation of dopamine at synapses

117. Beta-endorphin is

(1) a substance involved in perception of pain

(2) released from the pituitary in response to stress

(3) a neurotransmitter

(4) a peptide

118. When compared with the general population, relatives of persons who have bipolar affective disorder are more likely to display

(1) major depression

(2) phobic disorder

(3) cyclothymic personality

(4) obsessive compulsive personality

119. Evidence supporting the dopamine hypothesis of schizophrenia includes which of the following observations?

(1) Butyrophenones have molecular configurations similar to those of dopamine

(2) Thioxanthenes can produce parkinsonian side effects

(3) Phenothiazines block dopamine receptors

(4) Antipsychotic medications increase levels of dopamine metabolites

120. The actions of dextro-amphetamine (*d*-amphetamine) at catecholaminergic synapses include

(1) direct release of catecholamines into the synaptic cleft
(2) blockade of postsynaptic cate-cholamine receptors
(3) blockade of the catecholamine reuptake mechanism
(4) increased production of cate-cholamines through an increase in tyrosine hydroxylase

121. The Klüver-Bucy syndrome, produced in monkeys by bilateral temporal lobe lesioning, is characterized by

(1) compulsive oral activity
(2) rage attacks
(3) hypersexuality
(4) hypophagia

122. The principal dopaminergic pathway in the brain directly involves which of the following regions of the brain?

(1) Pontine raphe nuclei
(2) Putamen
(3) Locus ceruleus
(4) Substantia nigra

123. The right (nondominant) cerebral hemisphere is thought to mediate or control the function of

(1) visuospatial organization
(2) logical reasoning
(3) perception of body image
(4) quantitative ability

124. Persons treated with a mono-amine oxidase inhibitor, such as tranyl-cypromine sulfate (Parnate), for depression show an increase in the functional synaptic availability of

(1) acetylcholine
(2) serotonin
(3) histamine
(4) norepinephrine

DIRECTIONS: Each group of questions below consists of lettered headings followed by a set of numbered items. For each numbered item select the one lettered heading with which it is **most** closely associated. Each lettered heading may be used **once, more than once, or not at all.**

Questions 125–128

For each chemical classification, select the CNS neurotransmitter that is an example of that classification.

(A) Glutamic acid
(B) γ-Aminobutyric acid
(C) Norepinephrine
(D) Somatostatin
(E) Lactic acid

125. Biogenic amine

126. Excitatory amino acid

127. Neuropeptide

128. Inhibitory amino acid

Questions 129–133

For each function described below, select the hypothalamic nucleus most likely responsible.

(A) Anterior
(B) Ventromedial
(C) Lateral
(D) Posterior
(E) Supraoptic

129. Acts as a satiety center for appetite

130. Stimulates appetite

131. Functions with the reticular activating system to control arousal

132. Influences sexual behavior

133. Produces antidiuretic hormone

DIRECTIONS: Each group of questions below consists of four lettered headings followed by a set of numbered items. For each numbered item select

A	if the item is associated with	(A) only
B	if the item is associated with	(B) only
C	if the item is associated with	both (A) and (B)
D	if the item is associated with	neither (A) nor (B)

Each lettered heading may be used once, more than once, or not at all.

Questions 134–137

(A) Nonrapid eye movement (NREM) sleep
(B) Rapid eye movement (REM) sleep
(C) Both
(D) Neither

134. Functional enuresis (nocturnal type)

135. Penile erections

136. Dreaming

137. Distinctive electrographic features

Questions 138–141

(A) Dominant cerebral hemisphere
(B) Nondominant cerebral hemisphere
(C) Both
(D) Neither

138. Language

139. Hand preference

140. Linear, sequential, analytic information processing

141. Ataxia and intention tremor

Human Behavior: Biologic and Related Sciences

Answers

100.   The answer is C. *(Kaplan, ed 5. p 2.)* In the human brain, electrical impulses trigger chemical events. The release of presynaptic neurotransmitters stimulates postsynaptic receptors, allowing neuronal transmission to proceed. Synaptic communication between neurons is primarily chemical, which allows for the continuation of electrical impulses.

101.   The answer is B. *(Talbott, pp 16–20.)* The highest density of cholinergic innervation is found in the caudate nucleus and putamen. Acetylcholinesterase-reactive neuronal cell bodies located in the basal forebrain send cholinergic innervation to the cerebral cortex, hippocampus, and limbic structures. The locus ceruleus is the principal noradrenergic nucleus.

102.   The answer is C. *(Kaplan, ed 5. pp 39–41.)* Lesioning and stimulation studies have shown that the hypothalamus exerts control over sleep, appetite, and sexual and emotional behavior. Hypothalamic hormones and other blood-borne factors can influence behavior; moreover, the release and action of these substances are affected by the neurotransmitters—norepinephrine, serotonin, and dopamine—that mediate behavior. Memory is a complex function that involves cortical and subcortical structures and is affected by hypothalamic activity only in a secondary way.

103.   The answer is D. *(Michels, vol 3, chap 59, pp 1–5.)* Studies have reported that natural births are roughly a third more common at 3 AM than at 5 AM, and deaths 30 percent more common at 5 AM than at midnight. The timing of these events is thought to be directly related to biologic rhythm. Body temperature follows a 24-h rhythm, peaking at midafternoon. Depression has been linked to changes in the cortisol cycle. Personality disorders have not, to date, been linked to any biologic rhythm.

104.   The answer is C. *(Michels, vol 3, chap 60, pp 12–13.)* Although reports in the early 1960s suggested deprivation of REM sleep as a cause of psychosis and anxiety, this is no longer believed to be true. Deprivation of REM sleep has not been shown to cause any psychopathologic symptoms in recent sleep studies in fact, 50 percent of depressed patients "tested" with deprivation of REM sleep improved with no other treatment

105.   The answer is A. *(Kaplan, ed 5. p 1623. Michels, vol 3, chap 70, pp 1–13.)* Tardive dyskinesia is a repetitive involuntary muscle movement of the lips, tongue, jaw, neck, back, or extremities that is seen in some patients late in the course of treatment with antipsychotic medications. It often appears days to weeks after drug treatment is stopped. Its highest prevalence is in elderly females.

106.   The answer is D. *(Hales, pp 74–76.)* γ-Aminobutyric acid (GABA) is believed to be the major inhibitory neurotransmitter in the central nervous system. It has an important role in modulating the activity of other neurotransmitters. Many investigators believe that it has an important role in the etiology of anxiety disorders, though the exact mechanisms are still speculative.

107.   The answer is B. *(Michels, vol 2, chap 52, p 8.)* Cataplexy is the inability to carry out voluntary muscle movements while awake. It results from a sudden inhibition of muscle tone and varies from complete powerlessness to involvement of isolated muscle groups. It is frequently triggered by intense emotional states and lasts seconds to minutes. Neuroleptics are not used in its treatment.

108.   The answer is B. *(Hales, pp 192–193, 196.)* In 1939 Goldstein was the first to describe the catastrophic reaction, first noted with patients with brain disease. It consists of an emotional outburst that typically may involve anger, depression, tears, refusal, shouting, or sometimes aggressive behavior. This is in response to physical damage to the brain (reported more frequently among patients with left hemispheric lesions and aphasia) or as a psychological reaction to severe physical or cognitive impairment. These patients are typically angry or aggressive toward the examiner and the examination that is provoking the response.

109.   The answer is D. *(Kaplan, ed 5. pp 1610–1611.)* The amino acid tyrosine is the precursor in the synthesis of dopamine and norepinephrine. Tyrosine is converted to 3,4-dihydroxyphenylalanine (dopa), which is then decarboxylated to dopamine. Through the action of the enzyme dopamine-β-hydroxylase, dopamine is converted to norepinephrine. According to current biochemical theories, this pathway is of critical importance in the pathogenesis of depression.

110.   The answer is E. *(Hales, pp 213–214.)* Temporal lobe lesions are associated with symptoms that can mimic psychiatric illness. These symptoms include affective states (such as anger or depression), depersonalization, and memory impairment. Because olfactory or gustatory hallucinations are relatively rare in psychiatric disorders, their presence should suggest organic disease. Automatisms are complex, stereotyped behaviors carried out during psychomotor seizure activity.

111. The answer is E. *(Hales, pp 57-59.)* Neurotransmitters are chemical messengers that transfer information between neurons, i.e., from pre- to postsynaptic neurons. To be designated as a neurotransmitter, a substance must satisfy a number of criteria. These criteria include the necessity for a mechanism to inactivate the neurotransmitter after its release from the presynaptic nerve terminal. This is usually a catabolic enzyme system or an active reuptake mechanism.

112. The answer is E. *(Kaplan, ed 5. p 351.)* Prospective longitudinal studies are studies in which persons who are "vulnerable" (i.e., at high risk for psychiatric illness because of a positive family history) are identified at birth and followed over a period of time. Such studies are less subject to methodological bias than other approaches. For example, when compared with retrospective studies, prospective longitudinal studies tend to give a more accurate representation of early signs and symptoms of a given disorder and thus offer a better opportunity for the discovery of successful preventive approaches.

113. The answer is D. *(Hales, pp 56-57.)* Information is transmitted along a neuron by way of a bioelectrical process that is partially dependent on properties of the cell membrane. These properties result in a voltage difference being maintained across the membrane of an inactive neuron. Incoming stimuli depolarize the membrane, and if a threshold level is reached, an action potential is generated that reverses the polarity of the membrane. Propagation of the action potential down the axon, to its terminal button, causes the release of neurotransmitter into the synaptic cleft.

114. The answer is A. *(Hales, pp 57-59.)* Putative central nervous system neurotransmitters are generally classified in three groups: amino acids, biogenic amines, and neuropeptides. GABA is an inhibitory amino acid. The biogenic amines include the catecholamines (e.g., dopamine, norepinephrine, epinephrine), acetylcholine, histamine, and indolamines (e.g., serotonin). The neuropeptides include such substances as beta-endorphin, somatostatin, and vasopressin.

115. The answer is A (1, 2, 3). *(Kaplan, ed 5. pp 3-4.)* In determining the genetic influence in emotional disorders, a variety of research models have been employed. Following twins through their lives, particularly when they are identical twins, is the most common method. Most research centers maintain twin registries. Studies of adoptees are valuable in determining nature-versus-nurture issues, as are studies of familial risk. Drug responses are not used in determining genetic factors.

116. The answer is B (1, 3). *(Kaplan, ed 5. pp 919-920, 1627-1644.)* The woman described in the question most likely has a retarded depression and should have been treated with a tricyclic antidepressant. The exact mechanism of action of this class of medication is not known but is thought to involve inhibition of the reuptake of norepinephrine, dopamine, and serotonin. Recent studies also have shown that chronic administration of these drugs increases postsynaptic receptor sensitivity to norepinephrine and serotonin.

117. The answer is E (all). *(Talbott, pp 8–9.)* The endorphins are endogenous opioid peptides that are highly distributed in the brain. Their discovery led to the identification of a number of peptides that are thought to serve as neurotransmitters. Beta-endorphin has aroused considerable interest in psychiatry since it is released by the pituitary in response to stress and has an important role in perception of pain.

118. The answer is B (1, 3). *(Kaplan, ed 5. pp 880–881.)* Family studies of persons with documented bipolar affective disorders have shown a higher-than-expected frequency of relatives who have major depression or cyclic mood variation. In general, the morbidity is higher for relatives of persons with bipolar disease than for relatives of persons with unipolar disease. Family history of obsessive compulsive personality does not appear to affect morbidity in or increase the incidence of bipolar affective illness.

119. The answer is E (all). *(Kaplan, ed 5. pp 719–721.)* The hypothesis that schizophrenic symptoms are associated with abnormalities of dopamine metabolism is based on the fact that all effective antipsychotic medications block dopamine receptors. Such blockade results in increased production of dopamine (but decreased functional availability) and correspondingly increased levels of dopamine metabolites. Similarities in the molecular configurations of antipsychotic drugs and dopamine have been demonstrated by x-ray crystallography. Symptoms of Parkinson's disease, a disorder associated with dopamine deficiency in the brain, are produced as side effects of many antipsychotic medications.

120. The answer is B (1, 3). *(Kaplan, ed 5. pp 1612, 1831.)* Dextroamphetamine is a drug with mood-stimulating and appetite-suppressing properties. These properties are thought to be related to *d*-amphetamine's capacity to increase the synaptic availability of catecholamines by releasing them directly into synapses and by blocking their reuptake. The *dextro* isomer of amphetamine is three to four times as potent a stimulant of the central nervous as the *levo* isomer.

121. The answer is B (1, 3). *(Kaplan, ed 5. p 148.)* The Klüver-Bucy syndrome occurs in monkeys following bilateral temporal lobectomy involving the amygdala, the parahippocampal gyrus, the hippocampus, and the temporal cortex. It is a syndrome characterized by psychic blindness, compulsive oral activity, docility, hypersexuality, hyperphagia, and inability to ignore stimuli. Bilateral temporal lobe lesions in humans can produce modified versions of the same symptoms as well as severe memory loss.

122.   The answer is C (2, 4). *(Michels, vol 3, chap 44, pp 6–8.)* Neuroanatomic and neurochemical studies have revealed the presence of several dopaminergic pathways in the brain. The principal pathway has its origins in the substantia nigra and terminates in the caudate nucleus and putamen of the corpus striatum. Degeneration of this pathway causes the symptoms of Parkinson's disease. Other dopaminergic pathways originate in the cerebral cortex, arcuate nucleus of the hypothalamus, and in an area of the brain just dorsal to the interpeduncular nucleus.

123.   The answer is B (1, 3). *(Kaplan, ed 5. pp 149–155.)* Studies of persons with unilateral brain lesions as well as of persons who have had cerebral commissurotomies have suggested that the right cerebral hemisphere mediates certain nonverbal modes of perception and performance. In contrast to the left hemisphere, which is thought to control verbal, logical, and mathematical processes, the right hemisphere is thought to mediate visuospatial organization, perception of part-whole relationships, perception of rhythm, and integration of sensory and kinesthetic stimuli to form body images. Sex, age, and handedness can modify the asymmetry of cerebral hemispheric function.

124.   The answer is C (2, 4). *(Kaplan, ed 5. p 1651.)* Tranylcypromine sulfate (Parnate) is a member of the class of antidepressant drugs known as monoamine oxidase (MAO) inhibitors. Because the enzyme MAO is involved in the catabolism of both norepinephrine and serotonin, inhibition of this enzyme increases the availability of these neurotransmitters.

125–128.   The answers are: 125-C, 126-A, 127-D, 128-B. *(Hales, p 59.)* CNS neurotransmitters include amino acids, biogenic amines, and neuropeptides. There are many other neurotransmitter substances, and many are still poorly understood. This is one of the most exciting areas of current psychiatric research. As more and more knowledge accrues, it becomes possible to develop more specific psychopharmacologic interventions. The amino acids are excitatory (glutamic acid, aspartic acid) or inhibitory (GABA). The biogenic amines include the catecholamines such as dopamine, norepinephrine, and epinephrine. Other biogenic amines include acetylcholine, histamine, and the indolamine serotonin. There are numerous neuropeptides, including beta-endorphin, somatostatin, and vasopressin.

129–133.   The answers are: 129-B, 130-C, 131-D, 132-A, 133-E. *(Kaplan, ed 5. pp 40–41. Michels, vol 1, chap 28, p 7.)* The hypothalamus plays a central role in regulating a variety of psychologic functions that directly affect behavior and thus is key to the biologic expression of psychiatric illness. Sleep, appetite, and sexual and aggressive behavior are subject to its control. In addition, the hypothalamus regulates temperature, fluid balance, and pituitary function.

Through electrical stimulation and ablation studies, hypothalamic nuclei have been identified as having defined functions. The anterior nucleus appears to facilitate sexual interest and specific sexual behavior; lesions in this area eliminate the behavior. The ventromedial nucleus acts as a satiety center; stimulation of this area reduces appetite. The ventromedial nucleus exerts its control through inhibition of the lateral nucleus, which stimulates appetite. Ablation of the lateral nucleus results in fatal anorexia regardless of the state of the ventromedial nucleus. The posterior nucleus along with the contiguous reticular activating system controls the level of arousal; lesions in this area result in lethargy and somnolence. Aggression appears to be affected by stimulation of a number of different hypothalamic sites.

The hypothalamus also exerts control over the pituitary gland. The supraoptic and paraventricular hypothalamic nuclei produce vasopressin (antidiuretic hormone) and oxytocin, respectively. These hormones traverse the axons of their parent neurons to the posterior pituitary gland, from which they are released. The hypothalamus also produces a variety of releasing factors that control hormone secretion from the anterior pituitary gland.

134–137.   The answers are: 134-A, 135-B, 136-B, 137-C. (Talbott, pp 737–740, 749–750.) Sleep is commonly divided into REM and NREM periods. Each has typical and distinctive electrographic features. One will see differences on the electroencephalogram (EEG), the electro-oculogram (EOG), and the chin electromyogram (EMG).

There is considerable physiologic heterogeneity between REM and NREM sleep. During REM sleep both heart and respiratory rate, as well as blood pressure, tend to rise and show more variability than during NREM sleep. Skeletal muscle tone is less, and penile erections occur predictably in relation to REM sleep. When people are awakened from REM sleep, about 80 percent of the time they will report dreaming.

Sleepwalking, sleep terrors, and nocturnal functional enuresis are disorders of partial arousal out of the deepest levels of NREM sleep. They typically occur once nightly within the first several hours of sleep, and in most persons are "outgrown" by adolescence.

138–141.   The answers are: 138-A, 139-C, 140-A, 141-D. (Hales, p 4.) By definition, the dominant cerebral hemisphere is responsible for language. The left hemisphere is dominant in 97 percent of people, with the remainder showing either right hemispheric or mixed dominance. Hemispheric dominance and handedness are not synonymous, but they are usually closely related. For example, nearly all right-handed people have left hemispheric dominance for language. The two hemispheres have different styles of information processing. The dominant hemisphere processes information analytically in a sequential and linear fashion and does particularly well with processing language and symbolic information. The nondominant hemisphere processes language in a more gestalt or parallel fashion and does particularly well with visuospatial information. Most of the time the patient's preferred hand for writing will indicate language dominance. It can be confirmed by other demonstrations of handedness, such as pouring or cutting with a knife. Ataxia and intention tremor are signs of a cerebellar disorder.

Organic Mental Disorders and Consultation-Liaison Psychiatry

DIRECTIONS: Each question below contains five suggested responses. Select the one best response to each question.

142. All the following statements about complex partial seizures are true EXCEPT

(A) they are also known as psycho-motor or temporal lobe seizures
(B) impaired consciousness or loss of contact with the environment occurs
(C) the patient remembers associated automatisms as uncontrollable events
(D) associated automatisms can be ictal or postictal
(E) the focus is in temporal (limbic) structures

143. When assessing depression in the medically ill, which of the following symptoms is frequently the most diagnostic?

(A) Sleep disorder
(B) Poor appetite
(C) Low self-esteem
(D) Low energy level
(E) Decreased sex drive

144. Normal pressure hydrocephalus is usually associated with dementia, gait disturbance, and

(A) urinary incontinence
(B) seizures
(C) visual hallucinations
(D) auditory hallucinations
(E) aphasia

145. All the following statements about absence seizures are true EXCEPT

(A) they are also known as petit mal
(B) they are associated with an abrupt loss of attention to the environment
(C) the patient does not usually show confusion following the episode
(D) the loss of consciousness is usually for between 1 and 2 min
(E) during a seizure the patient may stare blankly or show automatisms such as lip smacking

Questions 146–148

A 22-year-old woman is admitted to the hospital because of right-hand anesthesia that developed after an argument with her brother. She is in good spirits and seems unconcerned about her problem. There is no history of physical trauma. The neurologic examination is negative except for reduced sensitivity to pain in a glove-like distribution over the right hand. Her entire family is in attendance and is expressing great concern and attentiveness. She ignores her brother and seems unaware of the chronic jealousy and rivalry described by her family.

146. The most likely diagnosis is

(A) body dysmorphic disorder
(B) histrionic personality disorder
(C) parietal brain tumor
(D) conversion disorder
(E) hysteria

147. The absence of anxiety in association with her lack of awareness of the psychological conflict with her brother is most likely due to

(A) marginal intellectual function
(B) hypochondriasis
(C) organic mental dysfunction
(D) primary gain
(E) psychosis

148. The patient's seeming enjoyment of the attention and concern of her family is most likely due to

(A) primary gain
(B) secondary gain
(C) tertiary gain
(D) indifference reaction
(E) suppression

149. The occurrence of delusions de novo in a person over the age of 5 years and without a known history of schizophrenia or delusional disorder should always alert the diagnostician to the possibility of

(A) agoraphobia
(B) frotteurism
(C) sleep disorder
(D) substance abuse
(E) dissociative disorder

150. Huntington's disease is associated with all the following EXCEPT

(A) autosomal dominant inheritance
(B) acute onset
(C) cerebral atrophy
(D) personality changes
(E) onset during adulthood

151. In which of the following age groups is the incidence of psychopathology the greatest?

(A) Under 10 years
(B) 10 to 25 years
(C) 25 to 45 years
(D) 45 to 65 years
(E) Over 65 years

152. A man given a placebo for mild pain reports 30 min later that the pain has resolved. The most appropriate conclusion is that the man

(A) has a conversion disorder
(B) has a dissociative disorder
(C) is malingering
(D) had no real pain to begin with
(E) responds to placebos

153. A 62-year-old woman is admitted to a medical unit because of an 11.4-kg (25-lb) weight loss over the last 3 months. She also reports anorexia, insomnia, fatigue, and decreased sexual interest. She does not have depressed affect and her mental status is judged to be unimpaired. Extensive medical evaluation is unremarkable. The most likely diagnosis is

(A) senile dementia
(B) occult malignancy
(C) hypochondriasis
(D) chronic anxiety
(E) masked depression

154. The most common cause of dementia in the elderly is

(A) multiple cerebral infarcts
(B) normal pressure hydrocephalus
(C) Alzheimer's disease
(D) Huntington's disease
(E) hardening of cerebral arteries

155. The sudden loss of muscular strength in association with laughter is most consistent with which of the following conditions?

(A) Catatonia
(B) Epilepsy
(C) Cataplexy
(D) Narcolepsy
(E) Hysteria

156. The condition known as "waxy flexibility" is encountered during the physical examination of patients with

(A) mania
(B) delirium tremens
(C) alcoholism
(D) hypochondriasis
(E) schizophrenia

157. Organic mental disorders typically are characterized by

(A) mental confusion, disorientation, and memory loss
(B) mental confusion, auditory hallucinations, and thought disorder
(C) depression, auditory hallucinations, and disorientation
(D) depression, visual hallucinations, and thought disorder
(E) depression, grandiosity, and sleep disorder

158. All the following statements about the condition known as obstructive sleep apnea are true EXCEPT that it is

(A) more common in men than in women
(B) more common in middle-aged adults than in children
(C) associated with excessive daytime hypervigilance
(D) often associated with snoring
(E) often associated with hypertension

159. According to the *Diagnostic and Statistical Manual of the American Psychiatric Association (DSM III-R)*, persons diagnosed with uncomplicated bereavement may display all the following EXCEPT

(A) a full depressive syndrome following loss of a loved one
(B) morbid preoccupation with general worthlessness
(C) guilt mainly about things done or not done near the time of death
(D) symptoms of insomnia and anorexia
(E) thoughts that he or she should have died with the deceased

160. The most common psychiatric disturbance associated with Cushing's syndrome is

(A) depression
(B) psychosis
(C) organic mental disorder
(D) mania
(E) anxiety neurosis

161. True statements regarding patients with Munchausen's syndrome include all the following EXCEPT

(A) they satisfy the *DSM III-R* criteria for factitious disorder
(B) they are usually motivated by the lure of disability income
(C) they have medical records in many hospitals and cities
(D) they are more often male than female
(E) they are characterized by pathologic lying

162. Which of the following prescribed medications has depression as a not-uncommon side effect?

(A) Insulin
(B) Prednisone
(C) Penicillin
(D) Imipramine (Tofranil)
(E) Tranylcypromine (Parnate)

163. True statements about post-cardiac surgery delirium include all the following EXCEPT

(A) it is the most common psychiatric complication of cardiac surgery
(B) it most commonly develops 2 to 4 days after surgery
(C) it is more common in dominant as opposed to dependent personalities
(D) it is more common in patients who express high preoperative anxiety
(E) it is more common in patients with a history of myocardial infarction

DIRECTIONS: Each question below contains four suggested responses of which **one or more** is correct. Select

A	if	**1, 2, and 3**	are correct
B	if	**1 and 3**	are correct
C	if	**2 and 4**	are correct
D	if	**4**	is correct
E	if	**1, 2, 3, and 4**	are correct

164. Symptoms commonly associated with premenstrual syndrome include

(1) irritability
(2) anxiety
(3) tension
(4) depression

165. Clinical observations of familial emotional responses in the premenstruum show that

(1) girls tend to repeat the symptom patterns of their mothers
(2) symptoms tend to peak in the fourth decade of life
(3) 5 to 10 percent of all women experience severe symptoms
(4) when daughters leave their mother's home, symptoms cease

166. Patients with organic mental syndromes commonly have symptoms involving

(1) behavior
(2) personality
(3) emotion
(4) cognition

167. The syndrome of delirium is usually characterized by

(1) inattention
(2) depressed affect
(3) clouded consciousness
(4) garrulousness

168. Correct statements about chronic subdural hematomas include which of the following?

(1) The majority are caused by head trauma
(2) The most common symptom is headache
(3) The symptoms may progress over days to weeks
(4) Fluctuations of consciousness predominate over any focal or lateralizing signs

169. The "epileptic personality" of patients with temporal lobe seizure commonly includes

(1) hyperreligiosity
(2) hypersexuality
(3) circumstantiality
(4) panic attacks

SUMMARY OF DIRECTIONS

A	B	C	D	E
1, 2, 3	1, 3	2, 4	4	All are
only	only	only	only	correct

Questions 170–172

A 52-year-old man presents with the chief complaint of feelings of hopelessness and helplessness, loss of interest, and poor sleep for the past 3 weeks. He is 25 lb overweight and smokes a pack of cigarettes a day. One month ago he was started on antihypertensives for his moderate hypertension of 150/95 mmHg. He reports being fired from his job of 18 years 6 weeks ago.

170. This patient's differential diagnosis should include

(1) adjustment disorder with depressed mood
(2) organic mood syndrome
(3) major depression
(4) dysthymia

171. Appropriate management of his hypertension should include

(1) a weight reduction program
(2) a reduction of salt intake
(3) a regular exercise program with smoking reduction
(4) a rechecking of his blood pressure

172. If this patient began complaining of impotence, the likely causes would include

(1) drug effect
(2) primary impotence
(3) stress
(4) penile steal syndrome

173. Psychiatric features of Addison's disease include

(1) depression
(2) memory impairment
(3) irritability
(4) psychosis

174. Cluster headaches tend to differ from migraine in that they

(1) have no known precipitants
(2) are more common in males than females
(3) are often associated with agitation and at times head banging
(4) display a very slow onset with a typical prodromal phase

175. Subcortical dementias include

(1) Huntington's disease
(2) Parkinson's disease
(3) Wilson's disease
(4) Alzheimer's disease

176. In primary degenerative dementia of the Alzheimer type

(1) the onset is abrupt
(2) the onset is usually after the age of 65 years
(3) the loss of intellectual abilities is limited to memory functions
(4) there are changes in personality and behavior

177. Acute intermittent porphyria is characterized clinically by which of the following?

(1) Abdominal pain
(2) Constipation
(3) Psychosis
(4) Neurologic deficits

178. Features that commonly distinguish multi-infarct dementia from dementia of the Alzheimer type include

(1) a stepwise deterioration in intellectual functioning ("patchy" deterioration)
(2) an abrupt onset
(3) focal neurologic signs and symptoms
(4) an absence of personality changes

179. The Kleine-Levin syndrome is a disorder characterized by

(1) periodic attacks of hypersomnolence
(2) an onset usually in adolescence
(3) gluttony and hypersexuality during the episode
(4) a higher incidence in males

180. Elisabeth Kübler-Ross has described five major phases that occur in a person's psychological adjustment to impending death. These stages include

(1) acceptance
(2) denial
(3) anger
(4) bargaining

181. Klüver-Bucy syndrome is a neurologic condition characterized by

(1) visual agnosia
(2) hypersexuality
(3) hyperorality
(4) unilateral deafness

182. True statements regarding the hyperventilation syndrome include that it

(1) is usually associated with severe anxiety
(2) may be caused by salicylism, fever, and pulmonary emboli
(3) is associated with respiratory alkalosis
(4) may induce paresthesias, numbness, and tetany

183. A 55-year-old man, who is taking lithium carbonate for manic-depressive illness, is admitted to a hospital because of cardiac disease. Which of the following therapeutic measures might be expected to increase the man's plasma lithium concentration even if his lithium dosage remains constant?

(1) Administration of digitalis
(2) Administration of a thiazide diuretic
(3) Administration of methyldopa
(4) Maintenance on a low-sodium diet

184. Patients with AIDS dementia complex (ADC) often present with

(1) cognitive abnormalities such as forgetfulness or confusion
(2) motor abnormalities such as loss of balance or leg weakness
(3) behavioral abnormalities such as apathy or depression
(4) acute psychotic delirium

DIRECTIONS: Each group of questions below consists of lettered headings followed by a set of numbered items. For each numbered item select the one lettered heading with which it is most closely associated. Each lettered heading may be used once, more than once, or not at all.

Questions 185-188

Match the following.

(A) Wernicke's encephalopathy
(B) Korsakoff's psychosis
(C) Huntington's disease
(D) Wilson's disease
(E) Creutzfeldt-Jakob disease

185. Rapidly progressive and fatal dementia with a usual age of onset in the forties or fifties

186. An abrupt onset with oculomotor disturbances, cerebellar ataxia, and mental confusion

187. A chronic condition that characteristically presents with confabulation and memory problems

188. A disorder characterized by choreiform movements and dementia, with an age of onset usually in the thirties

Questions 189-195

For each concept in "psychosomatic medicine" below, select the name that is most closely associated with it.

(A) Elisabeth Kübler-Ross
(B) Franz Alexander
(C) Sigmund Freud
(D) Wilhelm Reich
(E) Flanders Dunbar

189. Psychosomatic illnesses are associated with specific unresolved neurotic conflicts

190. There are seven psychosomatic illnesses: bronchial asthma, ulcerative colitis, rheumatoid arthritis, essential hypertension, peptic ulcer disease, neurodermatitis, and Graves' disease

191. Hysterical neurosis results from memories that have been repressed

192. Psychosomatic illnesses are characterized by specific personality traits

193. Persons experiencing life-threatening illness go through distinct stages of psychological adjustment

194. Psychoanalysis should address the underlying character type as well as symptoms

195. Hysterical (i.e., histrionic) personality is characterized by seductiveness, excitability, and superficial interpersonal relationships

DIRECTIONS: The group of questions below consists of four lettered headings followed by a set of numbered items. For each numbered item, select

A	if the item is associated with	(A) only
B	if the item is associated with	(B) only
C	if the item is associated with	both (A) and (B)
D	if the item is associated with	neither (A) nor (B)

Each lettered heading may be used **once, more than once, or not at all.**

Questions 196–198

(A) Premenstrual syndrome (PMS)
(B) Dysmenorrhea
(C) Both
(D) Neither

196. Symptoms most prominent in the late luteal phase

197. Antipsychotic medication indicated in treatment

198. Symptoms affected by diet and exercise

Organic Mental Disorders and Consultation-Liaison Psychiatry

Answers

142. The answer is C. *(Hales, pp 213-214.)* Impairment of consciousness is a hallmark of complex partial seizures. The focal discharge is associated with a temporal aura, and as this discharge spreads to the limbic system, impaired consciousness and loss of contact with the environment ensue. Automatisms are highly integrated, unconscious movements not remembered by the patient. They commonly include such activities as lip smacking, rubbing, running, disrobing, or the perseveration of acts initiated prior to loss of consciousness. Automatisms can be ictal or postictal events.

143. The answer is C. *(Michels, vol 2, chap 99, pp 1-7.)* Patients with medical illness can develop many of the vegetative signs of depression—for example, sleep problems, decreased appetite, low energy, and decreased sexual interest—as a result of being ill and in the hospital. In these patients the cognitive-affective symptoms, or how one feels about oneself, are commonly the most important diagnostic cues.

144. The answer is A. *(Hales, pp 270-271.)* Many dementias are chronic, slowly progressive, and unresponsive to treatment. One major exception is normal-pressure hydrocephalus. It is difficult to diagnose, but often is precipitated by such acute events as trauma, subarachnoid hemorrhage, or meningitis. Classically it is associated with gait ataxia and urinary incontinence. Headaches and papilledema are absent. Clinical improvement is sometimes dramatic when the cerebrospinal fluid is shunted away from the central nervous system into the cardiovascular system.

145. The answer is D. *(Hales, p 214.)* During an absence seizure, also called petit mal, the patient has an abrupt loss of attention while remaining awake and maintaining posture. The seizure activity rarely lasts beyond 20 s, and the patient displays an abrupt return of attention without residual confusion. Stereotyped or automatic behavior (such as lip smacking, chewing, or blinking) is common, but there is not a generalized convulsion. Some patients may show mild clonic, atonic, or tonic activity.

146–148. **The answers are: 146–D, 147–D, 148–B.** *(American Psychiatric Association, ed 3-R, pp 257-259. Hales, p 192.)* This patient displays some of the classic findings in conversion disorder. She has an alteration of physical functioning that suggests a physical disorder, the altered function was precipitated by a psychological event, the pattern (glovelike anesthesia) cannot readily be explained by a known disorder, and physical findings are negative. Patients with body dysmorphic disorder are preoccupied with imagined defects in their appearance, which is normal. The term *hysteria* is used pejoratively to mean that the symptoms are not real, but it is not an actual diagnosis. Patients with a parietal tumor would likely have other signs and symptoms.

The patient's lack of anxiety and awareness of the existence and significance of the conflict with her brother is a classic finding in conversion disorder. It is an example of "primary gain." This refers to keeping an internal conflict or need out of awareness, reducing the anxiety associated with it, and finding a partial solution to the underlying conflict. The enjoyment of attention from her family is an example of "secondary gain," which serves to reinforce the symptom. There is no such thing as "tertiary gain," and suppression refers to placing something into the preconscious rather than the unconscious. The indifference reaction is associated with right hemispheric lesions and consists of symptoms of indifference toward failures, lack of interest in family and friends, enjoyment of foolish jokes, and minimizing physical difficulties.

149. **The answer is D.** *(American Psychiatric Association, ed 3-R, pp 109-110.)* Schizophrenia and delusional disorder most often, but not always, first appear in persons under the age of 35 years. When delusions appear de novo without such a history, one must always consider the possibility of an organic delusional disorder. Abuses of substances such as cannabis, cocaine, amphetamines, and hallucinogens are common causes of organic delusional syndrome. Other causes include cerebral lesions and interictal phenomena in temporal lobe epilepsy.

150. **The answer is B.** *(Hales, pp 274-275.)* Huntington's disease is a rare illness that is inherited as an autosomal dominant trait and typically manifests during adulthood. It is characterized clinically by the insidious onset of choreiform movements, dementia, and personality changes. No effective treatment is presently known. At autopsy, the brain of affected persons is atrophied, especially in the caudate nucleus and putamen.

151. **The answer is E.** *(Kaplan, ed 5, pp 2014-2016.)* Persons older than 65 years of age have a higher risk than other persons of developing mental illness. However, elderly persons are underrepresented in the frequency of visits to mental-health clinics and in the receipt of appropriate social services. Common psychiatric problems in this population include depression and organic mental disorders.

152. The answer is E. *(Michels, vol 3, chap 45, pp 8–9.)* The only conclusion that can be reached about the man described in the question is that he responds to placebos. His response says nothing about whether his pain is "real" or psychogenic. Placebos have been shown to decrease pain of both psychological and physiologic origin.

153. The answer is E. *(Michels, vol 1, chap 59, p 12.)* Depressive illness consists of both somatic and psychological components. The somatic components include insomnia, anorexia, weight loss, fatigue, motor retardation or agitation, and decreased sexual interest. The psychological components include depressed mood, pessimism, and feelings of worthlessness and guilt. Not all components are present in every case. Patients who have a masked depression present with primarily somatic symptoms and few or no psychological ones. Diagnosis often is made only after extensive medical evaluation is unrevealing. The woman described in the question did not have any signs of dementia; medical evaluation did not reveal an organic disease process; and although hypochondriasis and chronic anxiety could have caused many of her symptoms, they are not likely to have caused the 11.4-kg weight loss.

154. The answer is C. *(Michels, vol 1, chap 73, pp 5–8.)* Although estimates vary, it is currently believed that 50 percent of demented elderly suffer from senile dementia of the Alzheimer type. The cause of this disorder is unknown and no treatment for it exists. Approximately 20 percent of demented elderly suffer from cerebral arteriosclerosis (previously described as hardening of the cerebral arteries). Cerebral arteriosclerosis produces dementia by causing multiple cerebral infarcts. Normal pressure hydrocephalus and Huntington's disease are rare causes of dementia.

155. The answer is C. *(Kaplan, ed 5. p 558.)* Cataplexy is the sudden and brief loss of muscular tone that occurs during the expression of a strong emotion. Affected persons remain conscious throughout each episode, which usually lasts no longer than 2 min. Cataplexy often occurs in patients with narcolepsy who may also have hypnagogic phenomena and sleep paralysis. The cause is unknown.

156. The answer is E. *(Kaplan, ed 5. pp 457, 578.)* Waxy flexibility is a condition in which patients will maintain, for long periods of time, postures into which they are placed. When one moves the patient's arms, one feels a resistance as if bending a wax rod. It is seen in catatonic patients and, therefore, in schizophrenia. Patients with mania and delirium tremens tend to be restless or hyperactive or both, and waxy flexibility is not seen in alcoholism or in hypochondriasis.

157. The answer is A. *(Kaplan, ed 5. pp 602–605.)* An organic mental disorder is characterized by disorientation, memory loss, mental confusion, and occasionally by visual hallucinations. The disorder occurs commonly in both medical and surgical patients and is often the result of metabolic abnormalities or adverse reactions to medication. When the disorder has an acute onset, reversible causes should be sought.

158. The answer is C. *(Talbott, pp 746-747.)* Sleep-disordered breathing is an important cause of persistent insomnia. It is more common in men than in women. The syndrome of obstructive sleep apnea is associated with excessive daytime sleepiness (not hypervigilance) and is often found in middle-aged, hypertensive, and overweight men. The bed partners of these patients complain bitterly about the patients' snoring.

159. The answer is B. *(American Psychiatric Association, ed 3-R. pp 361-362.)* The term *uncomplicated bereavement* is used to describe a normal reaction to the death of a loved one. Such an occurrence is frequently associated with a full depressive syndrome including poor appetite, weight loss, insomnia, and decreased libido. Marked functional impairment, marked psychomotor retardation, and morbid preoccupation with worthlessness suggest the possible development of a major depression. It is not at all unusual for such patients to express that they would be better off dead, or to wish they too had died.

160. The answer is A. *(Kaplan, ed 5. p 1211. Wilson, ed 12. p 1721.)* Cushing's syndrome often is associated with psychiatric disturbances. Depression is the most common disturbance and may range from moderate to severe; as many as 10 percent of affected persons attempt suicide. Mania, psychosis, and an organic mental disorder also can occur.

161. The answer is B. *(Talbott, pp 550-551.)* Patients with Munchausen's syndrome satisfy all the *DSM III-R* criteria for a factitious disorder with physical symptoms. In contrast to the other factitious disorders, Munchausen's syndrome is more common in males. The syndrome is characterized by pathologic lying, simulated and dramatic medical illness or self-mutilation, and a pattern of wandering from hospital to hospital. By definition, the factitious disorders, including Munchausen's syndrome, are motivated by a psychological need to assume the sick role and not by external incentives such as economic gain.

162. The answer is B. *(Kaplan, ed 5. p 1295.)* There are a number of drugs that not uncommonly are associated with the side effect of depression. These include adrenocortical steroids, such as cortisone and prednisone; estrogens and progestins, as are found in birth control pills; and thyroid medications. These drugs may cause depression directly or upon withdrawal. Penicillin is not associated with depression, and both imipramine (Tofranil) and tranylcypromine (Parnate) are used to treat depression.

163. The answer is D. *(Kaplan, ed 5. p 1323.)* Postcardiac surgery delirium is the most common psychiatric complication of cardiac surgery. While it may occur immediately, more commonly it follows a lucid period of 2 to 4 days. Patients with dominant personalities appear more likely to develop delirium, as do patients with low preoperative anxiety. This is probably due to difficulty in accepting the dependent sick role, while the denial of anxiety serves as an ineffective defense mechanism. Patients with a history of myocardial infarction are at higher risk probably because of cerebral anoxia secondary to diminished cardiac output.

164. The answer is E (all). *(Michels, vol 2, chap 120, p 2.)* There have been many physical and emotional symptoms associated with premenstrual syndrome (PMS). Irritability, tension, depression, and anxiety are among the most common. Physical symptoms include breast tenderness, abdominal bloating, and swelling of the ankles. Some researchers have attempted to cluster certain symptoms together in an attempt to delineate PMS subtypes. The reliability of this is questionable.

165. The answer is A (1, 2, 3). *(Michels, vol 2, chap 120, p 2.)* Clinical observation of menstrual responses in families has shown a tendency for girls to repeat the symptom patterns of their mothers. These do not change when leaving home. Symptoms of the premenstrual syndrome tend to peak in the fourth decade of life. It is estimated that approximately 5 to 10 percent of women in the United States experience severe menstrual symptoms.

166. The answer is E (all). *(Nicholi, pp 358-360.)* Patients with organic mental disorders often display defects of cognitive function. This is demonstrated on the mental status examination by difficulties with memory, calculation, language, and proverb interpretation. However, often there are also changes in noncognitive functions such as behavior, personality, and emotional regulation. Personality change and the appearance of lack of emotional control should always alert the clinician to the possibility of this diagnosis.

167. The answer is B (1, 3). *(Nicholi, pp 360-363.)* Delirious states usually have a sudden onset, often in the context of a medical illness. The most common finding is a defect in attention. This presents as an inability to concentrate, as well as distractibility. The patient is often unable to complete a coherent sentence and may misperceive distracting stimuli. Disorientation and memory loss may be present, but are not essential to the diagnosis. The disturbance of consciousness may extend from quietness and a tendency to fall asleep all the way to lethargy, stupor, or coma. Some patients display hypervigilance or agitation or have illusions or hallucinations.

168. The answer is E (all). *(Hales, pp 195-196. Wilson, ed 12. pp 2004-2006.)* Approximately 60 percent of chronic subdural hematomas follow head trauma. Other causes include ruptured aneurysms and rapid deceleration injuries. Headache is the most common symptom. As intracranial pressure gradually increases, one encounters signs associated with dementia. These include confusion, inattention, apathy, memory loss, drowsiness, and ultimately coma. Fluctuations in the level of consciousness predominate over focal or lateralizing neurologic signs, though such signs are not rare.

169.   The answer is B (1, 3). *(Hales, p 218.)* The so-called epileptic personality described for patients with temporal lobe seizures commonly includes hyper-religiosity, circumstantiality, and hypergraphia. These patients most commonly display hyposexuality. On the MMPI they often have elevations on the paranoia and schizophrenia scales. It is important to remember that all of these psychiatric manifestations can occur in other psychiatric disorders.

170-172.   The answers are: 170-A (1, 2, 3), 171-E (all), 172-B (1, 3). *(American Psychiatric Association, ed 3-R pp 112, 222-223, 232-233, 330-331.)* In assessing this patient's symptoms we find a significant stressor—losing a job of 18 years—which could account for an adjustment disorder. He is taking antihypertensive medication, which may be associated with the onset of depressive feelings (i.e., an organic mood syndrome). Since his dysphoria has lasted for longer than 2 weeks, and since he also has loss of interest in past pleasurable activities, as well as poor sleep, major depression cannot be ruled out. Dysthymia is not a consideration, since this diagnosis requires a 2-year history of depressive symptoms.

Nondrug measures used in the treatment of hypertension include relief of stress, dietary management, regular exercise, and control of other risk factors, such as cigarette smoking. Dietary management involves the restriction of sodium, cholesterol, and saturated fats, as well as the restriction of calories if the patient is overweight. Regular monitoring of blood pressure is indicated.

Male impotence, the inability to obtain or maintain an erection or the inability to achieve orgasm, can be brought on by a variety of biologic, psychological, or social causes. Antihypertensive medications are notorious for causing impotence, as is emotional stress. When a man has never had normal sexual functioning, this is defined as primary impotence. The penile steal syndrome occurs when blood is diverted from the penis to the gluteal region with resultant detumescence.

173.   The answer is E (all). *(Kaplan, ed 5. pp 1212-1213. Wilson, ed 12. pp 110-111.)* Addison's disease results from atrophy of the adrenal cortices. This may result from primary degeneration or be secondary to other diseases such as tuberculosis. The production of adrenal steroids is greatly diminished. Common psychiatric features include depression, apathy, anxiety, and irritability. Memory impairment may occur in as many as three-fourths of patients. Although rare, psychosis may also be present.

174.   The answer is A (1, 2, 3). *(Hales, pp 226-230.)* Cluster headaches share some similarities with migraine, but they also have some distinguishing features.

The female-to-male ratio is 2:3, as opposed to 3:1 for migraine. There are usually flurries of attacks, without a known precipitant. The onset is generally rapid and severe. Migraine usually has a more gradual onset, but both types of headache may be associated with nausea and vomiting. Migraine patients usually want to lie still, since movement aggravates their pain. Cluster headache patients are often agitated and may even bang their head in an effort to relieve pain.

175. The answer is A (1, 2, 3). *(Hales, pp 117–118.)* Subcortical dementias generally involve the basal ganglia, thalamus, and rostral brainstem structures. Because of this, these dementias have movement disorders as a prominent part of their symptoms. Typical examples include Huntington's disease, Parkinson's disease, and Wilson's disease. In contrast, Alzheimer's disease represents a type of cortical dementia that does not involve subcortical structures and does not manifest a movement disorder.

176. The answer is C (2, 4). *(American Psychiatric Association, ed 3-R, pp 119–120.)* In primary degenerative dementia of the Alzheimer type, there is an insidious onset with a progressive and deteriorating course. The dementia involves multiple areas of cognition, including memory, judgment, abstract thinking, and other higher cortical functions. There are often profound changes in personality and behavior as the disorder progresses.

177. The answer is E (all). *(Kaplan, ed 5. p 1294.)* Abdominal pain, constipation, neurologic deficits, and psychosis are all clinical features of acute intermittent porphyria. Although the course of the disease is extremely variable, initial presentation often consists of recurrent attacks of abdominal pain, with neurologic and emotional disturbances developing later. Attacks of the illness may be precipitated by medication, especially barbiturates. The diagnosis can be established by testing urine for porphobilinogen.

178. The answer is A (1, 2, 3). *(American Psychiatric Association, ed 3-R, pp 121–122.)* Multi-infarct dementia is due to cerebrovascular disease and is usually associated with focal neurologic signs and symptoms. The onset is typically abrupt, with a stepwise course that early on may leave some intellectual functions relatively intact. The deficits are "patchy" depending on which areas of the brain are damaged. In Alzheimer's dementia the onset is more gradual, and the course more uniformly progressive. Both conditions are associated with significant personality and behavioral changes.

179. The answer is E (all). *(Hales, p 253.)* Kleine-Levin syndrome is a disorder of sleep. It is characterized by periodic attacks of hypersomnolence and megaphasia. Most often it has an onset in adolescence, more commonly in males, but it may begin later in life. Hypersexuality and personality disturbances are also seen during episodes. Sleepiness may be as severe as that seen in narcolepsy or obstructive sleep apnea, and sleep studies often show multiple sleep-onset REM periods.

180. The answer is E (all). *(Kaplan, ed 5. pp 1340-1341.)* Elisabeth Kübler-Ross has described five phases of psychological adjustment that people pass through when confronted with the knowledge they are dying. Characteristically, the first stage involves denial of death and isolation of feelings. Affected persons then experience anger at their fate and may begin bargaining (often with God) in order to avert death. A period of depression finally is followed by acceptance. These responses do not necessarily occur in this sequence; several of them may occur simultaneously, or they may be mixed with other responses.

181. The answer is A (1, 2, 3). *(Kaplan, ed 5. p 148. Michels, vol 1, chap 28, p 8. Wilson, ed 12. p 201.)* The Klüver-Bucy syndrome is a behavioral syndrome that follows destructive lesions in both temporal lobes. Conditions that produce the syndrome include viral encephalitis, trauma, infarction, Pick's disease, and Alzheimer's disease. This behavioral syndrome is characterized by visual agnosia (e.g., inability to distinguish relatives from strangers), hypermetamorphosis (e.g., manual exploration of the environment), hyperorality (i.e., bulimia, or placing nonfood items in mouth), hypersexuality, aphasia, amnesia, and dementia. The hyperorality and hypersexuality may superficially resemble the behavior of patients who suffer from mania.

182. The answer is E (all). *(Talbott, pp 502-503.)* Hyperventilation leads to decreased arterial P_{CO_2}, increased pH, and resultant respiratory alkalosis. It is usually associated with severe anxiety. The cause may be anxiety or any medical condition that can produce hyperventilation. Such conditions include salicylism, fever, and pulmonary emboli. Patients usually complain of light-headedness, numbness around the lips, or tingling sensations in the extremities. Tetany occurs if the condition becomes severe.

183. The answer is C (2, 4). *(Kaplan, ed 5. pp 1661-1662.)* Lithium carbonate is eliminated from the body through urinary excretion. Both low-sodium diets and use of thiazide diuretics increase lithium concentrations in the plasma by increasing the reabsorption of lithium by the kidney. Thus, patients placed on either or both of these treatments should have their plasma concentration of lithium frequently monitored and the dosage of lithium adjusted accordingly to avoid toxicity.

184. The answer is E (all). *(Kaplan, ed 5. pp 1307-1309.)* The AIDS dementia complex (ADC) is a distinct syndrome, most probably caused by chronic encephalitis and myelitis due to human immunodeficiency virus (HIV). Patients may present acutely with a psychotic delirium, but more commonly they present with the typical clinical triad of motor, cognitive, and behavioral symptoms, which may be quite subtle in the early phase. Cognitive symptoms include forgetfulness, loss of concentration, and confusion. Behaviorally one often sees apathy, social withdrawal, and dysphoric mood. Loss of balance and leg weakness are common motor findings.

185-188. The answers are: 185-E, 186-A, 187-B, 188-C. *(Hales, pp 119, 149-152.)* Both Wernicke's and Korsakoff's syndromes are associated with thiamine deficiency, often resulting from alcoholism. Wernicke's encephalopathy has an abrupt onset with mental confusion, cerebellar ataxia, and oculomotor disturbances such as nystagmus or gaze palsy. The general confusional state may ultimately deteriorate, with the development of Korsakoff's psychosis and ultimately stupor and coma. Korsakoff's psychosis is chronic, with both retrograde and anterograde amnesia. Confabulation is common.

Creutzfeldt-Jakob disease may present with neurotic-like symptoms or as dementia and is fatal. It usually begins in the forties or fifties and rapidly progresses to severe dementia and death often in 1 year. It appears to be caused by a "slow" virus.

Wilson's disease is due to an inborn error of copper metabolism and usually has an onset in adolescence. The early onset with bizarre behavior and flattened affect may lead to a misdiagnosis of schizophrenia, although the neurologic signs usually precede the psychiatric symptoms. Not all cases show significant psychiatric symptoms.

Huntington's disease is a hereditary disorder that usually begins when the patient is in his or her late thirties. It is associated with choreiform movements and a progressive dementia that eventually, over decades, culminates in apathy and death.

189-195. The answers are: 189-B, 190-B, 191-C, 192-E, 193-A, 194-D, 195-D. *(Kaplan, ed 5. 356-360, 427-428, 1159-1161, 1340-1341.)* Sigmund Freud developed the concepts of psychological conflict and repression. He believed that persons who had hysterical neuroses suffered from the repression of memories and the feelings associated with them. His original ideas led to the development of psychoanalysis and laid the groundwork for psychosomatic medicine. Freud's early work was concerned mainly with symptoms.

Wilhelm Reich, a student of Freud, called attention to the importance of character types in diagnosis and treatment. One of the personality types he discussed was the hysterical personality, which he characterized as seductive, easily excitable, and superficial in interpersonal relationships.

Personality type and psychological conflict both have been cited as pathogenetic factors causing physical symptoms and psychosomatic illnesses. Flanders Dunbar thought that persons who had psychosomatic illnesses had specific personality traits. Franz Alexander gave major impetus to the concept that the seven classic psychosomatic illnesses—bronchial asthma, ulcerative colitis, rheumatoid arthritis, essential hypertension, peptic ulcer disease, neurodermatitis, and Graves' disease—were characterized by specific, unresolved neurotic conflicts. For example, he felt that persons with peptic ulcer disease had conflicts about oral dependency. Recent investigators, however, have questioned the specificity of his formulations, in part because many neurotic conflicts occur in association with more illnesses than the seven listed by Alexander. In fact, most—if not all—medical and surgical illnesses have concomitant psychological factors; in that sense, they are all psychosomatic in nature.

Elisabeth Kübler-Ross has written extensively on psychological adjustment to impending death.

196-198. The answers are: 196-A, 197-D, 198-C. *(Michels, vol 2, chap 120, pp 2-3.)* Premenstrual syndrome (PMS) is characterized by the onset of symptoms, both physical (breast tenderness, abdominal swelling) and emotional (irritability, depression, anxiety) in the late luteal phase, usually the week before the onset of menses. The patient is symptom-free during the first 2 weeks after her menstrual period starts. Dysmenorrhea is pain associated with the time of menstrual flow, usually the first 2 or 3 days. Mild analgesics, particularly nonsteroidal anti-inflammatory agents, are used for dysmenorrhea. Both conditions can be improved with exercise and dietary manipulation. PMS has responded to anxiolytics like alprazolam, but not antipsychotics.

Schizophrenia, Delusional, and Other Psychotic Disorders

DIRECTIONS: Each question below contains five suggested responses. Select the one best response to each question.

199. Which of the following statements regarding thought disorder is true?

(A) It is invariably found in schizophrenia
(B) It is sometimes exhibited by patients with mania
(C) It is one of the main criteria for the diagnosis of schizophrenia in the third edition of *Diagnostic and Statistical Manual of Mental Disorders (DSM III-R)*
(D) It is reflected in the speech but not the written communication of schizophrenics
(E) It is a phenomenon of schizophrenia first described by Sigmund Freud

200. Which of the following statements regarding delusions is true?

(A) Delusions are almost exclusively found in schizophrenia
(B) Delusions of grandiosity are rarely encountered except in mania
(C) Delusions involve a disturbance of cognition
(D) Delusions involve a disturbance of perception
(E) Delusions are a type of hallucination

201. All the following statements about patients with schizotypal personality disorder are true EXCEPT

(A) they often have bizarre modes of thought
(B) they are often eccentric in behavior
(C) they frequently become overtly schizophrenic as they get older
(D) they not uncommonly have relatives who are or were schizophrenic
(E) their communication is often unusual

Questions 202–203

202. Clozapine (Clozaril) is a recently introduced drug that has shown promise in the treatment of

(A) bipolar disorder
(B) recurrent major depression
(C) chronic schizophrenia
(D) Alzheimer's disease
(E) panic disorder

203. The side effects commonly associated with clozapine include all the following EXCEPT

(A) tardive dyskinesia
(B) sedation
(C) agranulocytosis
(D) hypersalivation
(E) seizures

204. Which of the following statements about visual hallucinations is true?

(A) They are more common than auditory hallucinations in schizophrenia
(B) They are almost always frightening to the patient
(C) They are more common in schizophrenia than in organic brain disorders
(D) They are a common occurrence in schizotypal personality disorder
(E) None of the above

205. Which of the following statements is true about the likelihood of relapse in the long-term treatment of schizophrenia with neuroleptic medication?

(A) Relapse is more likely with oral than injectable neuroleptics
(B) After 1 year the relapse rate is about one-third
(C) The relapse rate is higher in more intelligent patients
(D) Nearly all patients will relapse within 5 years
(E) None of the above

206. Which of the following drugs may induce a psychosis that is easily confused with, or misdiagnosed as, paranoid schizophrenia?

(A) Barbiturates
(B) Heroin
(C) Benzodiazepines
(D) Amphetamines
(E) Chlorpromazine

207. In the criteria set forth by *DSM III-R*, which of the following would distinguish schizophrenia from a manic episode?

(A) The schizophrenic patient will exhibit evidence of a thought disorder
(B) The manic patient is persistently elated, whereas the schizophrenic patient displays blunted, flat, or inappropriate affect
(C) The schizophrenic's psychosis is most often treated with neuroleptic medication
(D) The schizophrenic's psychosis is chronic while manic episodes are always intermittent
(E) None of the above

208. It has been demonstrated that lower socioeconomic status is associated with a higher prevalence rate for schizophrenia. True statements concerning this relationship include all the following EXCEPT

(A) it has been attributed to the effects of downward social mobility secondary to the illness
(B) it has been attributed to social and health conditions within lower socioeconomic environments
(C) it is supported by prevalence rates two or more times higher than those found in higher socioeconomic groups
(D) it is supported by the finding that the prevalence rate is higher in immigrant populations
(E) it has been demonstrated within the United States, but not within Europe

209. Correct statements regarding the diagnostic criteria for delusional (paranoid) disorder, according to *DSM III-R*, include all the following EXCEPT

(A) auditory or visual hallucinations, if present, are not prominent
(B) behavior is not bizarre
(C) delusions are bizarre
(D) any associated affective syndrome is of brief duration relative to the duration of the delusional disturbance
(E) an organic factor has not initiated and maintained the disturbance

210. The lifetime risk for suicide in schizophrenic patients is estimated to be approximately

(A) 0.5 percent
(B) 3 percent
(C) 10 percent
(D) 25 percent
(E) 35 percent

211. Studies of the relationship between gender and schizophrenia have generally demonstrated that

(A) the usual age of onset is earlier for females than males
(B) males tend to have a better prognosis than females
(C) the lifetime risk of developing schizophrenia is approximately the same in males and females
(D) males tend to respond better to neuroleptic medication
(E) there is a higher concordance rate in male monozygotic twins as compared with female monozygotic twins

212. The mental status examination of patients with schizophrenia most commonly demonstrates a marked disorder of

(A) orientation
(B) memory
(C) mood
(D) thinking
(E) insight

213. The diagnosis of schizoaffective disorder includes all the following EXCEPT

(A) the condition does not meet the criteria for schizophrenia

(B) the condition does not meet the criteria for mood disorder

(C) the patient has presented with both schizophrenic psychotic symptoms and a mood disturbance, and at other times with psychotic symptoms without mood symptoms

(D) during an episode there have been delusions or hallucinations for at least 2 days but less than 2 weeks

(E) no organic factor initiated or maintained the disturbance

DIRECTIONS: Each question below contains four suggested responses of which one or more is correct. Select

A	if	**1, 2, and 3**	are correct
B	if	**1 and 3**	are correct
C	if	**2 and 4**	are correct
D	if	**4**	is correct
E	if	**1, 2, 3, and 4**	are correct

214. True statements about the course and prognosis of schizophrenia include which of the following?

(1) Some schizophrenic illnesses will resolve completely and never recur even without treatment

(2) Outcome has improved considerably in the last 50 years

(3) Catatonic and hebephrenic forms have become less frequent

(4) Research suggests that an initial onset following a stressful event may be associated with a better prognosis

215. True statements about the occurrence of thought disorder include which of the following?

(1) Bleuler considered it the most important characteristic of schizophrenia

(2) It occurs frequently in schizophrenia and affective disorders

(3) Its presence may cause manic patients to be misdiagnosed as schizophrenic

(4) It disappears when the patient is no longer actively psychotic

216. The *DSM III-R* criteria for schizophreniform disorder include

(1) all the psychotic symptom criteria for schizophrenia except for duration

(2) schizophrenic-like symptoms caused by hallucinogens

(3) an illness that lasts less than 6 months

(4) severe affective symptoms with thought disorder but no other signs of schizophrenia

217. Correct statements regarding paranoid disorders include that they

(1) are more common than schizophrenia

(2) are associated with delusions that are usually less bizarre and fragmented than in schizophrenia

(3) are associated with delusions of persecution, but not of jealousy

(4) usually are not associated with Schneiderian first-rank symptoms

218. The use of neuroleptics to manage and treat schizophrenia may be associated with which of the following side effects?

(1) Acute dystonia

(2) Gynecomastia

(3) Parkinsonism

(4) Galactorrhea

219. Signs or symptoms more likely to be associated with the catatonic type of schizophrenia than with other subtypes include

(1) neologisms
(2) psychomotor disturbance
(3) word salad
(4) excitement and stupor

220. Correct statements about malignant neuroleptic syndrome include that it is

(1) believed to result from blockade of dopamine receptors in the brain
(2) characterized by severe autonomic and extrapyramidal dysfunction
(3) associated with hyperthermia
(4) usually fatal

221. Some researchers have divided symptoms of schizophrenia into negative and positive. Negative symptoms include

(1) hallucinations
(2) blunted affect
(3) delusions
(4) social withdrawal

DIRECTIONS: Each group of questions below consists of lettered headings followed by a set of numbered items. For each numbered item select the **one** lettered heading with which it is **most** closely associated. Each lettered heading may be used **once, more than once, or not at all.**

Questions 222-225

Match the following.

(A) Emil Kraepelin
(B) Eugen Bleuler
(C) Harry Stack Sullivan
(D) Frieda Fromm-Reichman
(E) Sigmund Freud

222. The schizophrenogenic mother

223. Dementia praecox renamed *schizophrenia*

224. Interpersonal theory of schizophrenia

225. The symptoms of schizophrenia (dementia praecox) delineated on the basis of course and outcome

Questions 226-229

For each major preoccupation or experience related to body function, select the most likely diagnosis.

(A) Koro
(B) Delusional disorder
(C) Body dysmorphic disorder
(D) Delirium tremens
(E) Schizophreniform disorder

226. The conviction that parasites are crawling within the skin, but general behavior not obviously odd or bizarre

227. Belief that one's genitals are being retracted into the body

228. Visions involving extraterrestrials using a weapon to shoot parasites into the body, which causes unbearable itching

229. Frightening visual hallucinations of being attacked by bugs in a patient with a clouded sensorium

Schizophrenia, Delusional, and Other Psychotic Disorders

Answers

199. The answer is B. *(Michels, vol 1, chap 53, pp 9-12.)* The abnormalities found in schizophrenic speech and writing were originally best described by Kraepelin and Bleuler. While these were originally considered to be a hallmark of that illness, modern investigation and clinical experience have shown that they can also be exhibited by patients with other psychiatric disorders, such as mania. Thought disorder is commonly found in schizophrenia, but there are significant numbers of patients who do not demonstrate the phenomenon. *DSM III-R* recognizes that a disturbance in thinking is but one of a number of criteria that are necessary to make the diagnosis.

200. The answer is C. *(Talbott, p 365.)* Delusions are found in a wide variety of psychotic conditions other than schizophrenia, including organic disorders and some mood disorders. A delusion is defined as a firmly held belief that is untrue and contrary to a person's educational and cultural background. The patient clings to the belief even in the face of great contrary evidence. The delusions of schizophrenia show a wide variety of themes, but no particular theme is specific to either schizophrenia or any other mental disorder. While grandiose delusions are a common finding in mania, they are also found in other conditions. Hallucinations are disorders of perception.

201. The answer is C. *(American Psychiatric Association, ed 3-R, pp 340-342.)* Peculiar and *eccentric* are the words most often used to describe persons with a schizotypal personality disorder. This includes their speech patterns, ideation, appearance, and the way they relate to others. The content of their thought may include paranoid suspiciousness and ideas of reference (though not delusions), as well as odd or magical beliefs or fantasies (though not hallucinations, loosening of associations, or incoherence). They rarely have close friends and are very anxious in social situations. Schizotypal personality disorder is differentiated from schizophrenia by the absence of any protracted period of psychosis and failure to display a true formal thought disorder. The disorder is believed to be more common among the first-degree biologic relatives of people with schizophrenia than among the general population.

202-203. The answers are: 202-C, 203-A. *(Kaplan, ed 5. pp 1610, 1626.)* Clozapine (Clozaril) is a recently introduced and approved drug that has shown promise in the treatment of chronically and severely ill schizophrenic patients. This includes some patients who have failed to respond to standard antipsychotic medication. Improvement has been noted in both positive and negative symptoms. Because 1 to 2 percent of patients may develop agranulocytosis, a potentially fatal disorder, a structured weekly monitoring system has been developed. Another potentially severe side effect is seizure, which affects, depending on dosage, up to 5 percent of patients. Other common problems include sedation, hypersalivation, tachycardia, constipation, and effects on blood pressure. The drug does not seem to produce extrapyramidal side effects, and the absence of reported tardive dyskinesia has been of great interest. Longer experience with the drug will be necessary to determine fully the profile of side effects.

204. The answer is E. *(Talbott, pp 364–365.)* Visual hallucinations are not at all common to schizophrenia, and when they are encountered the clinician should always seriously consider the possibility of an organic brain syndrome. While visual hallucinations may certainly be frightening to the patient, they may also be relatively neutral or pleasurable. When visual hallucinations are present in schizophrenia they are usually as common during the day as during the night, whereas in organic brain disorders they are more common at night. Auditory hallucinations are highly characteristic of schizophrenia, but can also occur in organic brain disorders.

205. The answer is B. *(Kaplan, ed 5. pp 787–792.)* While reported results vary widely, over the past 2 decades most studies suggest that about one-third of schizophrenic patients will have a recurrence of their psychosis despite maintenance on neuroleptic medication. Such medication clearly reduces, but does not eliminate, the risk of relapse. Relapse rates have been similar even in studies in which compliance is controlled through the use of longitudinal injectable medication. There are significant numbers of patients who do not relapse when followed over many years. The decision for long-term drug maintenance therapy is a complex one that must weigh benefits versus the risk of serious side effects.

206. The answer is D. *(Nicholi, pp 270–271.)* Abuse of amphetamines can result in a psychosis very closely resembling acute paranoid schizophrenia. Symptoms include paranoid delusions and visual hallucinations. Some investigators feel that prominent visual hallucinations and a relative absence of thought disorder are more characteristic of amphetamine psychosis, but other investigators feel the symptoms are indistinguishable. Other drugs that produce psychoses similar to schizophrenia include phencyclidine (PCP) and lysergic acid diethylamide (LSD).

207. The answer is E. *(American Psychiatric Association, ed 3-R pp 192–195, 216–218. Talbott, pp 360–362.)* None of the distinctions set forth in this question apply to the disorders. An affective diagnosis may be associated with "first rank" symptoms su̇ ᶦ as thought broadcasting or thought insertion; and similarly, the presence of mood-incongruent delusions or hallucinations, in the absence of a full affective syndrome, may point toward schizophrenia. While it is true that in schizophrenia there must be continuous signs of illness for at least 6 months, this need not be continuous psychosis but may include prodromal or residual symptoms. Mania is usually episodic, but chronicity of psychosis does not exclude the diagnosis of mania if other criteria are fulfilled. It is true that most often mania is treated by lithium, but neuroleptic medication is commonly used with both schizophrenia and the acute phases of mania. Also, treatment methodology is not part of the diagnostic criteria.

208. The answer is E. *(Talbott, pp 381–382.)* Higher incidence and prevalence of schizophrenia have been found repeatedly to occur in association with lower socioeconomic conditions, whether urban or rural. The evidence is more striking in large urban centers. This has been demonstrated both in Europe and the United States. Depending upon the study, the incidence has been reported to be as much as six times higher in lower socioeconomic groups. Some feel this relationship is causal—that it is due to such factors as social isolation, poor prenatal care, and the stress of poverty. There is probably better evidence for the hypothesis that the relationship is due to downward social drift as a consequence of the impaired motivation, social skills, cognition, and employability secondary to the illness.

209. The answer is C. *(American Psychiatric Association, ed 3-R pp 201–202.)* The delusions in delusional (paranoid) disorder are not bizarre. This fact helps to differentiate the condition from paranoid schizophrenia or schizophreniform disorder, in which delusions are usually bizarre and hallucinations are often present. In delusional disorder the delusions usually involve situations that occur in real life, such as being followed, poisoned, loved at a distance, and so on.

210. The answer is C. *(Stoudemire, pp 220–221.)* The lifetime risk for suicide in schizophrenic patients is estimated at 10 percent. This is somewhat less than is the case for mood disorders. Alcoholics have a similar lifetime risk, estimated at 12 percent.

211. The answer is C. *(Kaplan, ed 5. pp 717–718.)* Gender differences in schizophrenia have been repeatedly demonstrated. The lifetime risk for schizophrenia is the same in males and females, but males tend to have an earlier peak age of onset (18 to 25 years versus 26 to 45 years for females) and a poorer outcome. Females appear to be more responsive to neuroleptics, and in monozygotic twin studies the concordance rates are higher in females than in males.

212. The answer is D. *(American Psychiatric Association, ed 3-R pp 187–190.)* The most common clinical finding during the mental status examination of a patient with schizophrenia is the presence of a thinking disorder. This may be a disorder of thought processes or content or both. Common findings include looseness of associations, autistic thinking, a failure of the ability to abstract, and delusional ideation. One certainly can encounter disturbances of mood and a lack of insight, but these are not hallmark features of the diagnosis. When cognition and memory disturbances seem to be present, they are usually secondary to the patient's agitation, autism, and thought disorder.

213. The answer is D. *(American Psychiatric Association, ed 3-R pp 209–210.)* The diagnosis of schizoaffective disorder is one of the most confusing and controversial in psychiatric nosology. It is considered when the condition does not meet the criteria for either schizophrenia or mood disorder but the patient at one time has presented with symptoms of both, and, at another time, with psychotic symptoms without mood symptoms. During an episode of the disturbance, the delusions or hallucinations must have been present for at least 2 weeks in the absence of prominent mood symptoms.

214. The answer is E (all). *(Michels, vol 1, chap 53, pp 16–18.)* The outcome of schizophrenic illnesses is very variable, and it has long been known that some will resolve completely, with or without treatment. Other patients will have repeated recurrences, with either full or partial recovery between episodes. Still other patients will show a relentless downhill course. It is clear that prognosis has improved over the years, presumably as a result of better treatment. Paranoid forms of the disorder have become more common, while catatonic and hebephrenic illnesses are less common. A number of studies have demonstrated that there are characteristics of the initial illness that are more likely to be associated with a good prognosis. These include an acute onset following stress, confusion or perplexity, and prominent affective symptoms. However, if schizophrenia is defined as in *DSM III-R*, it may be that these "good prognosis" patients were suffering with affective or schizophreniform disorders.

215. The answer is A (1, 2, 3). *(Talbott, p 365.)* While thought disorder was regarded as the salient symptom of schizophrenia by Bleuler, research has clearly demonstrated that it also occurs in manic and depressive patients. The tangential looseness of associations (derailment) and illogicality of manic patients is also common in schizophrenic patients. There is no specific thought disorder that is exclusively found in schizophrenia. Often the thought disorder will lessen or disappear with the resolution of the active psychosis, but this is by no means a certainty. The thought disorder may continue to be evident even during remission.

216. The answer is B (1, 3). *(Michels, vol , chap 70, pp 8–10.)* DSM III-R criteria for schizophreniform disorder meet all the criteria for schizophrenia, except that the duration is less than 6 months. This includes all phases of the disorder, including the prodromal and residual phases. It probably includes many of the cases of "good prognosis schizophrenia" that were described in many early studies of prognosis. By definition these patients do not include those with sufficient affective symptoms to be diagnosed as having an affective disorder, nor patients with drug-induced or other organic psychoses.

217. The answer is C (2, 4). (*Michels, vol 1, chap 68, pp 1-15.*) Paranoid disorders are associated with psychosis that includes persistent delusions of persecution or of jealousy, but lacks the criteria for a diagnosis of schizophrenia, affective disorder, brief reactive disorders, or organic mental disorder. The delusions are typically more "tightly organized" and less bizarre and fragmented than in schizophrenia. It must be remembered that paranoid symptoms may be associated with organic mental disorder, such as that produced by use of amphetamines.

218. The answer is E (all). (*Michels, vol 1, chap 55, pp 20-26.*) Neuroleptic medication is associated with a wide variety of potential side effects. The antidopaminergic drugs may produce a number of extrapyramidal movement disorders, such as dystonias, parkinsonism, tardive dyskinesia, and akathisia. They may also elevate prolactin levels, which may result in gynecomastia, galactorrhea, and sexual and menstrual dysfunction. Another serious side effect is the potentially fatal malignant neuroleptic syndrome.

219. The answer is C (2, 4). (*American Psychiatric Association, ed 3-R, p 196.*) The essential feature of the catatonic type of schizophrenia is psychomotor disturbance. This may present as stupor, negativism, posturing, rigidity, or excitement. Mutism is common, as is alteration between extreme excitement and stupor. The condition is now relatively rare.

220. The answer is A (1, 2, 3). (*Michels, vol 1, chap 55, p 25.*) Malignant neuroleptic syndrome is a very serious side effect of treatment with neuroleptic medication. It is potentially fatal, with a mortality that approaches 20 percent. Typically there is severe autonomic and extrapyramidal dysfunction, altered consciousness, and hyperthermia. Laboratory findings include leukocytosis and elevated creatine phosphokinase. An early diagnosis and discontinuance of neuroleptics are essential. The response to drugs such as bromocriptine mesylate has suggested that dopamine receptor antagonism is associated with this disorder.

221. The answer is C (2, 4). (*American Psychiatric Association, ed 3-R, pp 187-198.*) *Schizophrenia* is a term used to represent a group of mental disorders that include such symptoms as delusions, hallucinations, and formal thought disorder. These disorders usually have an onset by early adulthood, though sometimes much later, and may be associated with a deterioration of functioning over time. Some researchers have divided symptoms into positive and negative. Positive symptoms, such as hallucinations and delusions, usually respond to antipsychotic medications. Negative symptoms, such as blunted affect and social withdrawal, are less consistently responsive.

222-225.   The answers are: 222-D, 223-B, 224-C, 225-A. *(Talbott, pp 358-360, 380-381.)* Emil Kraepelin (1828-1899) carefully studied the course and outcome of seriously mentally ill patients. He noted that some had symptoms such as delusions and withdrawal at a relatively early age and were likely to have a chronic and deteriorating course. To distinguish these patients with "dementia" at an early age from those with late-onset dementias, Alzheimer's disease, and manic depressive illness, he referred to the disorder as *dementia praecox.*

Bleuler (1857-1939) also observed patients over long periods of time and became convinced that a thought disorder, involving a "splitting" of cognitive functions, was the pathognomonic feature of this disorder. He renamed the condition *schizophrenia.*

Sigmund Freud felt that these patients were untreatable by psychoanalysis because of their severe libidinal regression, which made them unable to form relationships and, in particular, a transference.

Sullivan saw schizophrenia not so much in intrapsychic terms, but as a result of environmental influence in which the patient had an insufficient developmental exposure to positive interpersonal relationships.

Fromm-Reichman believed that schizophrenia was the outcome of an inadequate mother-child relationship in which the mother was aloof, overly protective, or hostile.

226-229.   The answers are: 226-B, 227-A, 228-E, 229-D. *(American Psychiatric Association, ed 3-R, pp 131, 199-203, 207-208. Kaplan, ed 5. p 845.)* Koro is a condition reported mainly in China, Malaysia, and Thailand that involves intense anxiety that one's genitals are retracting into the body. Males may attach devices to the penis to prevent the retraction, and females are concerned with the vulva or breasts. The patient believes that if the genitals become fully retracted into the abdomen, he or she will die.

Delusions involving bugs are common to a number of psychiatric disorders. Bizarre bodily delusions, in the absence of an organic disorder, most commonly are associated with the diagnosis of schizophrenia or schizophreniform disorder. The latter has features identical to those of schizophrenia, but the duration is less than 6 months.

Prominent hallucinations are not present in delusional (paranoid) disorder, and the general behavior is not obviously odd or bizarre. Patients with the somatic type of delusional disorder usually consult nonpsychiatric physicians for treatment of their perceived somatic condition.

Alcohol withdrawal delirium (delirium tremens) by definition is associated with global cognitive impairment and is often associated with vivid hallucinations, delusions, and agitated behavior. Global cognitive impairment is not found in the other conditions discussed above.

Body dysmorphic disorder involves preoccupation, not delusion.

Mood Disorders

DIRECTIONS: Each question below contains five suggested responses. Select the **one best** response to each question.

230. While the majority of women do not experience significant side effects when taking oral contraceptives, for those who do, the most commonly encountered psychological problem is.

(A) anxiety
(B) depression
(C) night terrors
(D) short-term memory defects
(E) long-term memory defects

231. Studies of bipolar illness show an average concordance rate in monozygotic twins of

(A) 10 percent
(B) 25 percent
(C) 50 percent
(D) 75 percent
(E) 95 percent

232. The occurrence of depression, as an early symptom, has been particularly associated with carcinoma of the

(A) prostate
(B) bladder
(C) parathyroid
(D) pancreas
(E) ovary

Questions 233–234

One month after the death of his father, a 27-year-old graduate student, with no prior psychiatric history, experiences the onset of irritability, difficulty concentrating, sudden fits of crying, and difficulty falling asleep.

233. The most likely diagnosis would be

(A) major depression
(B) dysthymia
(C) uncomplicated bereavement
(D) dependent personality disorder
(E) posttraumatic stress disorder

234. The most generally accepted initial treatment for this man's condition would be

(A) antidepressant medication
(B) neuroleptic medication
(C) psychoanalysis
(D) long-term psychodynamic psychotherapy
(E) brief supportive psychotherapy

235. A 27-year-old woman seeks evaluation for her "depression" in an outpatient clinic. She reports episodic feelings of sadness since adolescence. Occasionally she feels good, but these periods seldom last more than 2 weeks. She is able to work but thinks she is not doing as well as she should. In describing her problems she seems to focus more on repeated disappointments in her life and her low opinion of herself than on discrete depressive symptoms. In your differential diagnosis at this point, the most likely diagnosis is

(A) major depression with melancholia
(B) adjustment disorder with depressed mood
(C) cyclothymia
(D) childhood depression
(E) dysthymia

236. The cognitive functioning of a person with a major depression is often characterized by all the following manifestations EXCEPT

(A) bizarre associations
(B) suicidal ideation
(C) obsessive rumination
(D) concentration impairment
(E) memory impairment

237. The basis for the therapeutic effect of electroconvulsive therapy (ECT) is

(A) seizure activity
(B) electrical stimulation of the brain
(C) memory loss
(D) the depressed patient's wish for punishment
(E) the depressed patient's attitude toward ECT

238. All the following statements about postpartum depression and "maternity blues" are true EXCEPT

(A) postpartum depression occurs in 10 to 15 percent of all new mothers
(B) "maternity blues" occur in 50 to 80 percent of all new mothers
(C) postpartum depression is differentiated from "maternity blues" by persistence beyond the first 3 days following delivery
(D) the signs and symptoms of postpartum depression may be similar to those of a major depressive episode
(E) the treatment of postpartum depression is similar to that for major depression

239. Among seriously depressed patients, the proportion that can be expected eventually to commit suicide is

(A) less than 1 percent
(B) about 2 percent
(C) about 15 percent
(D) about 30 percent
(E) about 60 percent

240. All the following statements about suicide are true EXCEPT

(A) it is among the top ten leading causes of death in the United States
(B) it is almost always associated with illness, especially depression
(C) it has a significant familial incidence
(D) it is more apt to be completed in males than in females
(E) it is less likely in persons who have communicated their intent to others

241. While delusions of any variety can occur in major depressive disorder with psychotic features, the most common delusions are

(A) mood-incongruent
(B) mood-congruent
(C) mood-unrelated
(D) mood-controlling
(E) none of the above

242. A diagnosis of bipolar disorder might be appropriate for patients who have all the following EXCEPT

(A) recurrent depressions and a history of mania
(B) recurrent depressions without a history of mania
(C) mania now and a history of a depressive episode
(D) mania now without a history of past affective disturbances
(E) a history of several manic episodes without depression

243. According to *DSM III-R*, all the following characteristics are found in the melancholic type of major depressive episode EXCEPT

(A) typically worse depression in the evening
(B) early morning awakening
(C) psychomotor retardation or agitation
(D) significant anorexia or weight loss
(E) loss of interest or pleasure in all or most activities

244. True statements about depression that occurs concomitantly with a medical illness include all the following EXCEPT

(A) it may be the result of medication
(B) it is usually unresponsive to antidepressant medication
(C) it may not be related to the medical illness
(D) it may be the first symptom of the medical illness to appear
(E) it may have the same signs and symptoms as endogenous depression

245. Which of the following disorders is an absolute contraindication to the use of electroconvulsive therapy (ECT)?

(A) Aortic aneurysm
(B) Brain tumor
(C) Coronary artery disease
(D) Pregnancy
(E) None of the above

246. The concept that psychopathology, including depression, is the result of developmental deficits related to self-esteem and the development of a cohesive self is associated with the psychoanalyst

(A) Franz Alexander
(B) Carl Jung
(C) Harry Stack Sullivan
(D) Heinz Kohut
(E) Sigmund Freud

247. The term *double depression* is used to describe:

(A) a particularly severe bout of major depression
(B) major depression superimposed on dysthymia
(C) recurrent episodes of major depression within a 2-month period
(D) medical illness with a superimposed episode of major depression
(E) major depression superimposed on "maternity blues"

248. According to *DSM III-R*, all the following are criteria for a diagnosis of recurrent major depression EXCEPT

(A) there must have been at least two major depressive episodes
(B) recurrent major depressive episodes must have been separated by a period of at least 1 year of more or less usual functioning
(C) the current episode need not meet the full criteria for a major depressive episode if there has been a previous major depressive episode
(D) there has never been a manic episode
(E) there has never been an unequivocal hypomanic episode

249. True statements about seasonal affective disorder include all the following EXCEPT

(A) it is more common in women than in men
(B) it may be associated with mood elevation
(C) symptoms often include hypersomnia and weight gain
(D) it is commonly treated with light therapy
(E) depression characteristically begins in the fall or winter

250. True statements about disturbance of sleep associated with mood disorders include all the following EXCEPT

(A) patients often complain of early morning awakening
(B) depressed patients with bipolar illness often complain of excessive sleep
(C) sleep latency (time from sleep onset to REM sleep) is often reduced
(D) sleep deprivation may induce a temporary remission of depression
(E) manic patients generally require excessive amounts of sleep because of their hyperactivity

251. All the following statements about bipolar disorder are true EXCEPT

(A) the essential feature is one or more manic episodes usually accompanied by one or more major depressive episodes

(B) the initial episode that occasions hospitalization is usually depression

(C) there may be two or more complete cycles within a year

(D) mixed or rapidly cycling bipolar disorder tends to have a more chronic course than other types

(E) the disorder is equally common in males and females

DIRECTIONS: Each question below contains four suggested responses of which one or more is correct. Select

A	if	1, 2, and 3	are correct
B	if	1 and 3	are correct
C	if	2 and 4	are correct
D	if	4	is correct
E	if	1, 2, 3, and 4	are correct

252. The list of symptoms specified by DSM III-R for the diagnosis of a major depressive episode includes

(1) sleep disturbance
(2) loss of interest or pleasure
(3) significant weight loss
(4) depressed mood

253. Flight of ideas is a thought process characterized by

    rapid speech
(2) abrupt topic changes
(3) punning or plays on words
(4) goal-directed thought

254. The DSM III-R criteria for a major depressive episode specify that delusions or hallucinations

(1) must be mood-incongruent
(2) must not be present as a major symptom
(3) must be primarily associated with guilt feelings
(4) must not have been present for 2 weeks or more in the absence of prominent mood symptoms

255. According to DSM III-R, the criteria for a diagnosis of cyclothymia include

(1) a chronic mood disturbance of at least 2 years' duration
(2) numerous manic episodes and periods of depressed mood
(3) a 2-year period in which the person is never without the required symptoms for more than 2 months
(4) an onset in adolescence

256. According to DSM III-R, the criteria required for the diagnosis of dysthymia (depressive neurosis) include which of the following?

(1) Depressed mood most of the time for at least 2 years
(2) Symptoms while depressed that can include poor appetite, overeating, and low energy or fatigue
(3) No absence of a depressed mood for more than 2 months during a 2-year period
(4) No evidence of a major depressive episode during the first 2 years of the disturbance

DIRECTIONS: The group of questions below consists of lettered headings followed by a set of numbered items. For each numbered item select the one lettered heading with which it is most closely associated. Each lettered heading may be used once, more than once, or not at all.

Questions 257-260

Each statement listed below refers to an etiologic theory of depression. Select the name most closely associated with each statement.

(A) Kraepelin
(B) Lewinsohn
(C) Abraham
(D) Beck
(E) Seligman

257. In contrast to the usual mourner's grief over the lost person, the depressed person is concerned with loss and guilt resulting from unconscious hostility toward the lost person

258. Depression results from specific cognitive distortions present in depression-prone people

259. Depression relates to "learned helplessness"

260. The depressed person lacks social skills, and a decrease in pleasant events or an increase in unpleasant events leads to dysphoria and self-blame, which are then reinforced by the environment

DIRECTIONS: The group of questions below consists of four lettered headings followed by a set of numbered items. For each numbered item select

A	if the item is associated with	(A) only
B	if the item is associated with	(B) only
C	if the item is associated with	both (A) and (B)
D	if the item is associated with	neither (A) nor (B)

Each lettered heading may be used **once, more than once, or not at all.**

Questions 261-265

(A) Melancholic major depression
(B) Manic episode
(C) Both
(D) Neither

261. Irritability

262. Predominant sadness, hopelessness

263. Grandiose ideas

264. History of schizophrenia

265. Decreased sexual drive

Mood Disorders

Answers

230. The answer is B. *(Stoudemire, p 625.)* A great many studies have been done to determine the side effects of oral contraceptives, and the results are somewhat inconsistent. Most, however, suggest that the majority of women have no significant side effects. Many, but not all, studies report an increased incidence of depression.

231. The answer is D. *(Michels, vol 1, chap 62, pp 14–15.)* The evidence for a genetic factor in bipolar affective disorders is reasonably sound. The concordance rate for bipolar illness in monozygotic twins averages 80 percent, when various studies are combined. The concordance rate in dizygotic twins and siblings is 29 percent, which is significantly higher than that found in the general population.

232. The answer is D. *(Stoudemire, p 579.)* Carcinoma of the pancreas has long been associated with the occurrence of emotional disorder, and the most commonly described symptoms are depression and an intense sense of dread. The incidence of depression that predates the discovery of the malignancy varies from 10 to 50 percent. The symptoms are often similar to those of a major depressive episode, with or without vegetative signs.

233–234. The answers are: 233-C, 234-E. *(American Psychiatric Association, ed 3-R pp 247, 361–362. Michels, vol 1, chap 67, pp 8–10.)* Following the loss of a loved one, a full depressive syndrome can occur as a normal reaction. It usually occurs during the first 2 or 3 months following the loss. It is distinguished from major depression by the absence of morbid preoccupation with worthlessness, prolonged and marked functional impairment, and marked psychomotor retardation. The absence of a previous history of chronic mood disorder would rule out the diagnosis of dysthymia. Posttraumatic stress disorder can be associated with depressive symptomatology, but by definition the condition follows a stressor event that is outside the range of usual human experience, such as simple bereavement. Personality disorders are not precipitated by a stressor event.

The treatment of a grief reaction is based on the presumption that it is a normal process, usually of brief duration. Any situation that provides grieving people a chance to express their feelings can be quite supportive. Family and friends usually provide this function. When disturbing symptoms cause a professional to be consulted, brief supportive psychotherapy would be the most common initial intervention. Drugs or long-term treatment approaches would usually be employed only with evidence of underlying psychopathology or the development of a psychiatric disorder.

235. The answer is E. *(American Psychiatric Association, ed 3-R, pp 230–233.)* Dysthymia is a chronic depression lasting more than 2 years, usually beginning in late adolescence or early adulthood. Sometimes patients describe being depressed for as long as they can remember. Symptoms fluctuate but are usually not severe. Such patients are commonly concerned with their perceived failures or interpersonal disappointments. The somatic symptoms characteristic of major depression or melancholia are less prominent in dysthymia.

236. The answer is A. *(Kaplan, ed 5, pp 896–902.)* People with typical unipolar depression ruminate about guilt, suicide, somatic fears, or other depressive themes. Concentration and recent-memory impairment, which at first may suggest an organic brain syndrome, improve with the lifting of depression. Concentration and memory difficulties that are secondary to the depression also may be difficult to distinguish from the side effects of antidepressant medication; thus, these symptoms should be carefully assessed before initiation of pharmacotherapy. Although the content of depressive thinking may be delusional or gruesome, the associations or connections characterizing the thought processes of depressed persons are usually conventional and seldom bizarre.

237. The answer is A. *(Kaplan, ed 5. pp 1675–1676.)* The therapeutic effect of ECT depends on the production of a seizure. (In fact, convulsions have a beneficial effect on depression, whether they are induced electrically or with medication.) Subconvulsive electrical stimuli can produce loss of consciousness and memory and may even meet a person's wish for punishment, but these results have no effect on the lifting of depression.

238. The answer is C. *(Stoudemire, pp 636–638.)* Approximately 50 to 80 percent of new mothers will experience "maternity blues" within the first week after delivery, usually resolving within 2 to 3 weeks. When the symptoms persist beyond the first postpartum month, and especially when the symptoms are particularly severe, a postpartum depression must be considered. It appears to occur in about 10 to 15 percent of new mothers, the symptoms are quite similar to those of major depression, and it is treated in a similar fashion.

239. The answer is C. *(Talbott, p 404.)* Suicide is an ever-present danger in seriously depressed persons. The clinician must constantly be on the alert for the signs and symptoms of potential suicide, even in patients who appear to be responding to treatment. It is estimated that approximately 15 percent of seriously depressed persons will eventually kill themselves.

240. **The answer is E.** *(Talbott, pp 1021-1033.)* Suicide is the ninth leading cause of death in the United States and is most often preventable. The vast majority of victims suffer from psychiatric illness, and the most common is mood disorder. Mood disorder has been identified in 40 to 80 percent of a consecutive series of suicides, and alcoholism in 20 to 30 percent. Males tend to be more successful than females in their attempts, and there is a clear familial association. It is estimated that up to 80 percent of suicide victims have communicated their intent to others, and thus such communications must be taken very seriously.

241. **The answer is B.** *(American Psychiatric Association, ed 3-R, p 220.)* When delusions or hallucinations are present in major depressive disorder, the delusional content is usually congruent with the patient's mood. Since patients with major depression are often filled with guilt and feelings of worthlessness, it is not surprising that their delusions most commonly involve persecution because of some moral transgression or inadequacy. Other mood-congruent delusions encountered are nihilistic or somatic delusions and delusions of poverty. Mood-incongruent delusions are less common. When present, they are often persecutory but with the patient unable to explain why they should be so treated.

242. **The answer is B.** *(American Psychiatric Association, ed 3-R, p 225. Kaplan, ed 5. pp 892-894, 907-909.)* The bipolar-unipolar distinction is made entirely on the basis of mania. A current manic episode or a history of mania establishes the diagnosis of bipolar disorder. The bipolar category is classified as depressed, manic, or mixed depending on the clinical presentation. The term *unipolar* is not part of official classification but is used by some clinicians for recurrent major depression.

243. **The answer is A.** *(American Psychiatric Association, ed 3-R, p 224.)* In the melancholic type of major depression, the patient typically complains of feeling worse in the morning. This is often associated with early morning awakening. As the day progresses, some patients will report a reduction in their feelings of depression.

244. **The answer is B.** *(Michels, vol 2, chap 99, pp 1-7.)* While it is true that depression may be the first manifestation of a medical illness, it is equally true that the discovery of a medical illness does not necessarily explain the genesis of the depression. On a symptom basis, depression secondary to medical illness is often indistinguishable from primary depression. The treatment of medical illness may be a primary cause of depression, as for example, depression secondary to steroid medication. Depression may also occur secondary to the consequences of the illness, for example, loss of autonomy and self-esteem or negative effects on personal and vocational life. When there are symptoms of a major depression, most patients will have a favorable response to the use of antidepressants.

245. The answer is E. *(American Psychiatric Association, Treatments. pp 1805-1806.)* There is no absolute contraindication to the use of ECT, but there are a number of conditions in which important risk factors must be weighed against the danger of untreated depression or depression unresponsive to treatment. The literature sometimes describes brain tumor to be an absolute contraindication because of the risk of brainstem herniation from increased intracranial pressure. However, there is growing evidence that with proper technique and medical management, these patients can safely undergo ECT. Bradycardia, tachycardia, hypertension, and increased cardiac work may occur during a seizure, and this may require modification in anesthetic technique to minimize the risk to patients with aneurysm or heart disease. A small series of case reports of ECT during pregnancy suggests that the procedure can be carried out with safety for both the mother and the fetus.

246. The answer is D. *(Talbott, p 142. Whybrow, pp 81-92.)* Heinz Kohut, originally a classical analyst, ultimately developed a theory of psychopathology emphasizing developmental deficit, as opposed to fixation and regression related to conflict regarding sexual and aggressive drives. He believed that the most important line of development related to the self, and especially to self-esteem and self-cohesion. The development of a cohesive self requires phase-appropriate empathy, in the form of mirroring and idealization from important objects ("selfobjects").

247. The answer is B. *(American Psychiatric Association, ed 3-R. p 229.)* Patients with dysthymia may develop a major depression. When they do, this is sometimes referred to as *double depression*. Such patients are at greater risk for having a recurrence of a major depressive episode than are those patients who have major depression only.

248. The answer is B. *(American Psychiatric Association, ed 3-R pp 228-230.)* All the statements specify diagnostic criteria for recurrent major depression, except for the statement regarding a symptom-free period. The criteria in *DSM III-R* state that there must be a period of at least 2 months between major depressive episodes, during which the patient returns to more or less usual functioning. It is estimated that about 50 percent of persons who initially have a single episode will eventually have another. People with recurrent major depression are also at greater risk for developing bipolar disorder than are those with a single episode.

249. The answer is B. *(American Psychiatric Association, Treatments. pp 1891-1892.)* Seasonal affective disorder has been recognized for quite some time, but the syndrome has been systematically investigated only in recent years. Patients are predominantly women, often with the depression and hypomania that has been associated with bipolar II disorder. The characteristic pattern is depression beginning in the fall and ending in the spring, often followed by euthymia, hypomania, or mania in the spring or summer. The depressive symptoms are often similar to those described by patients with atypical depression or bipolar illness, such as hypersomnia, carbohydrate craving, lack of energy, and weight gain. The common symptoms of depression—including hopelessness, depressed mood, and functional impairment—also occur.

250. The answer is E. *(Talbott, p 421.)* There is an important relationship between depression and sleep disturbance. In major depression, sleep studies have shown a number of changes, including a shortened sleep latency and a shift of REM sleep such that more occurs in the earlier part of the night. Depressed patients almost always have sleep complaints, and these include difficulty in failing asleep, intermittent awakening, and early morning awakening. Patients with atypical depression or bipolar disorder typically display hypersomnia, but their sleep is not described as restful. During mania patients do not seem to require a normal amount of sleep and may describe going for long periods without sleep. Sleep deprivation has been shown to be capable of inducing a temporary remission in both major depression and bipolar disorder.

251. The answer is B. *(American Psychiatric Association, ed 3-R. pp 225–226.)* Bipolar disorder occurs in about 0.4 to 1.2 percent of the adult population and is equally common in males and females. In the typical case, the initial episode is manic rather than depressed. The periods of disturbance in this disorder tend to be more frequent than the episodes of depression in recurrent major depression. The time intervals between episodes in bipolar disorder are variable, but the so-called rapid cyclers tend to have a more chronic course.

252. The answer is E (all). *(American Psychiatric Association, ed 3-R. p 222–223.)* All the named symptoms are among those for which *DSM III-R* require that at least five be present for the diagnosis of major depressive episode. Other specified symptoms include psychomotor agitation or retardation, fatigue or loss of energy, feelings of worthlessness or excessive/inappropriate guilt, diminished ability to think or concentrate, and recurrent thoughts of death or suicide. The criteria specify, however, that at least one of the symptoms must be either depressed mood or loss of interest/pleasure. The depressed mood should be present most of the day, nearly every day; and the loss of interest or pleasure should be in most activities and most of the time. In both instances these criteria can be met by either the subjective account of the patient or by the observations of others.

253. The answer is A (1, 2, 3). *(American Psychiatric Association, ed 3-R. p 215.)* Flight of ideas, a primary sign of mania, is a train of thoughts that is rapid and pressured. Although manic persons displaying flight of ideas usually lose sight of the original goal or point of their thoughts, the actual associations from one thought to the next are usually understandable and often are clever or humorous. In contrast, the thought associations of schizophrenic persons are more frequently bizarre and incomprehensible. In severe manic psychosis, associations may also become incomprehensible and speech disorganized.

254. The answer is D (4). *(American Psychiatric Association, ed 3-R p 223.)* Delusions and hallucinations may be associated with the diagnosis of a major depressive episode, but they are not required for the diagnosis. Often, but not always, they are associated with feelings of worthlessness or inappropriate or excessive guilt. Delusions or hallucinations must not have been present for more than 2 weeks prior to the development of mood symptoms, or after the mood symptoms have remitted. This helps to differentiate major depression from other psychoses that may have associated mood symptoms.

255. The answer is B (1, 3). *(American Psychiatric Association, ed 3-R pp 226-228.)* The essential feature of cyclothymia is a chronic mood disturbance of at least 2 years' duration (1 year for children and adolescents), during which there are numerous hypomanic episodes and periods of depressed mood or loss of interest or pleasure. However, the symptoms must not be of sufficient severity or duration to meet the criteria for major depressive or manic episodes. The affected person must never be without the required symptoms for more than 2 months in a 2-year period (1 year for children and adolescents). The diagnosis cannot be made if the disturbance is superimposed on another chronic psychotic disorder, such as schizophrenia, or maintained by an organic factor or substance abuse. Some investigators believe that this is a mild form of bipolar disorder. While the age of onset is usually in adolescence or early adulthood, it can occur either earlier or later. A particular age of onset is not one of the diagnostic requirements.

256. The answer is E (all). *(American Psychiatric Association, ed 3-R pp 230-233.)* All the factors listed are part of the *DSM III-R* criteria for a diagnosis of dysthymia. Of the specific symptoms listed in choice 2, only two need to be present during the period of depression. The list also includes insomnia or hypersomnia, low self-esteem, poor concentration, difficulty in making decisions, and feelings of hopelessness. In children and adolescents the requirement is modified such that the depressed mood must not be absent for more than 2 months during a 1-year period. The patient may still have this diagnosis if there was a previous major depressive episode more than 2 years before the disturbance, as long as there was a full remission such that there were no signs or symptoms for at least 6 months. If a major depression develops after a 2-year period of dysthymia, both diagnoses are given. Additional requirements for this diagnosis include an absence of any previous manic or hypomanic episodes and that the disturbance not be superimposed on chronic psychotic disorder. Also, it cannot be initiated or maintained by an organic factor, for example, the prolonged administration of an antihypertensive medication.

257-260.   The answers are: 257-C, 258-D, 259-E, 260-B. *(Talbott, pp 405, 424-427.)* Kraepelin was a pioneer in the classification of psychiatric disorders early in this century. He emphasized the longitudinal history and pattern of symptoms. He differentiated what he called manic-depressive illness (major depression, bipolar disorder, and some patients with dysthymia) from dementia praecox (schizophrenia). He noted that the former had an episodic and relatively benign course, while the latter was often chronic and deteriorating.

Abraham (1911) was an early psychoanalytic theorist who noted that unlike the usual mourner who grieves, the depressed person is preoccupied with guilt, loss, and inadequacy that are based on unconscious hostility toward the lost person. Freud (1917) expanded on these theories to note that, unlike the usual mourner, the depressed person is unable to resolve these ambivalent feelings. The anger toward the lost person is turned inward, resulting in dysphoria, guilt, and loss of self-esteem.

Lewinsohn (1974) proposed that the person who is likely to become depressed is one who lacks social skills. A subsequent decrease in response-contingent positive reinforcement (a decrease in pleasant events or an increase in unpleasant events) then leads to dysphoria and self-blame. Once the depression begins, the secondary gain (positive reinforcement from sympathy, attention, and so on) escalates the condition to the level of clinical depression.

Aaron Beck (1972) proposed a cognitive-behavioral model of depression. Depression-prone people have specific cognitive distortions ("depressogenic schemata") derived from early experience. These disturbed cognitions result in unrealistically negative views of self, world, and future.

Seligman proposed that experiences with uncontrollable events lead to cognitive and emotional deficits that result in a state of "learned-helplessness." The resultant expectations and conclusions about self and life events can result in depression.

261-265.   The answers are: 261-C, 262-A, 263-B, 264-D, 265-A. *(American Psychiatric Association, ed 3-R, pp 214-224.)* Melancholic depression and mania are both major affective disorders. Melancholia includes clinical manifestations such as irritability, severe sadness, anhedonia, crying, hopelessness, helplessness, impaired memory, pessimism, delusions of inadequacy or punishment, suicidal thoughts, social withdrawal, and decreased sex drive. It is not associated with a history of schizophrenia.

Mania, or the manic phase of bipolar affective disorder, is characterized by a euphoric, expansive mood state. Like melancholia, irritability is common, as is poor concentration. These patients are easily distractible, have flight of ideas, and express grandiose thoughts. They are uninhibited and show an increased sex drive. The mood is typically labile. Although sometimes misdiagnosed as schizophrenia, there is no relationship.

Anxiety, Somatoform, and Dissociative Disorders

DIRECTIONS: Each question below contains five suggested responses. Select the **one best** response to each question.

266. Which of the following statements most correctly describes panic disorder?

(A) When associated with agoraphobia, it occurs more often in males than females
(B) No increased familial incidence has been identified
(C) The usual age of onset is in young adulthood
(D) It is often relieved by anxiolytic medications but not by antidepressants
(E) It often requires hospitalization for the initial phase of treatment

267. All the following statements about agoraphobia are true EXCEPT

(A) it is more common in females
(B) it is rarely accompanied by panic disorder
(C) it may result in the patient's being totally housebound
(D) it is frequently associated with a fear of being alone
(E) it often has an onset between 20 and 30 years of age

268. All the following are true statements about multiple personality disorder EXCEPT

(A) the onset is usually in childhood
(B) there is often a history of childhood abuse
(C) the disorder is more common in females
(D) only one personality recurrently takes full control of the person's behavior
(E) the transition from one personality to another is usually sudden

269. All the following statements about generalized anxiety disorder are true EXCEPT

(A) there is persistent anxiety lasting for at least 1 month
(B) the disorder is equally common in females and males
(C) the onset is usually in young adulthood
(D) symptoms include vigilance and scanning
(E) mild depressive symptoms are common

270. True statements about obsessive compulsive disorder include all the following EXCEPT

(A) the onset is usually in adolescence or early adulthood
(B) patients attempt to neutralize thoughts or impulses by other thoughts or action
(C) anxiety is accentuated when a compulsion is carried out
(D) the disorder is found equally in men and women
(E) patients usually experience their compulsions or obsessions as intrusive and irrational

271. True statements about hyperventilation syndrome include all the following EXCEPT

(A) it may lead to respiratory acidosis
(B) it may produce a drop in serum calcium
(C) it is often associated with panic disorder
(D) it is associated with peripheral vasoconstriction
(E) it can be symptomatically reproduced by an infusion of sodium lactate

272. All the following statements about sleep panic are true EXCEPT

(A) it is a common complaint in patients with panic disorder
(B) it occurs as the result of dreams during REM sleep
(C) the symptoms are usually similar to those of daytime panic
(D) sleep deprivation may worsen the associated panic disorder
(E) REM latency is not reduced as it is in depressed patients

273. Which of the following statements regarding multiple personality disorder is true?

(A) Other psychiatric symptoms or diagnoses are rarely coexistent
(B) It is more common in men than women
(C) There is often a history of having been abused in childhood
(D) It usually begins in young adulthood
(E) It often occurs in several generations of the same family

274. All the following types of drugs are commonly used to treat anxiety states EXCEPT

(A) tricyclic antidepressants
(B) neuroleptics
(C) benzodiazepines
(D) monamine oxidase inhibitors
(E) beta-receptor blocking agents

275. Which of the following statements is true about the antianxiety drug buspirone (BuSpar)?

(A) It is a benzodiazepine
(B) It is particularly useful for the rapid treatment of acute anxiety states
(C) It is the most sedating of the commonly used antianxiety drugs
(D) On a per-milligram basis it is three times more potent than diazepam
(E) It has less potential for abuse than diazepam

276. All the following statements about pheochromocytoma tumors are true EXCEPT

(A) they may cause panic similar to spontaneous panic attacks
(B) they secrete catecholamines
(C) patients with pheochromocytoma rarely develop agoraphobia
(D) they are associated with malignant hypertensive episodes
(E) during an acute episode, patients generally demonstrate increased motor activity secondary to anxiety

277. Which of the following statements is true about postconcussional amnesia in contrast to dissociative (hysterical) amnesia?

(A) Postconcussional amnesia does not occur in combination with hysterical amnesia
(B) The retrograde amnesia following concussion generally does not extend beyond 1 week
(C) When postconcussional amnesia disappears, it does so rapidly and completely
(D) Hypnosis will commonly restore the lost memories of postconcussional amnesia
(E) None of the above

278. According to DSM III-R, the diagnosis of hypochondriasis requires that the disorder have a duration of at least

(A) 1 month
(B) 3 months
(C) 6 months
(D) 1 year
(E) 3 years

279. All the following are true statements about depersonalization disorder EXCEPT

(A) reality testing remains intact during the depersonalization experience
(B) patients express the sense of being detached from their mental processes or body, or of being in a dream-like state
(C) in the majority of patients it has a very slow and insidious onset
(D) it must be distinguished from occasional depersonalization, which is common and not necessarily pathologic
(E) it must be distinguished from depersonalization secondary to brain tumor or temporal lobe epilepsy

DIRECTIONS: Each question below contains four suggested responses of which one or more is correct. Select

A	if	**1, 2, and 3**	are correct
B	if	**1 and 3**	are correct
C	if	**2 and 4**	are correct
D	if	**4**	is correct
E	if	**1, 2, 3, and 4**	are correct

280. As a consequence of panic disorder, the patient may develop

(1) generalized anxiety
(2) secondary depression
(3) agoraphobia
(4) psychosis

281. Which of the following can cause symptoms similar to those found in panic disorder?

(1) Pheochromocytoma
(2) Hypoglycemia
(3) Intoxication with caffeine
(4) Withdrawal from barbiturates

282. The locus ceruleus theory for the etiology of panic attacks is supported by the observation that

(1) yohimbine provokes anxiety
(2) electrical stimulation of the locus ceruleus produces anxiety
(3) tricyclic antidepressants may block panic attacks
(4) sodium lactate provokes anxiety in patients without panic disorder

283. Alcoholic amnestic disorder is distinguished from psychogenic amnesia by which of the following statements?

(1) Short-term, but not immediate, memory is impaired
(2) There is lack of awareness of impairment of memory
(3) Confabulation is common
(4) Blunted affect is common

284. While the differentiation of anxiety from depression is often difficult, generally patients with generalized anxiety disorder

(1) do not demonstrate the full range of vegetative symptoms seen in depression
(2) do not respond to treatment with tricyclic antidepressants
(3) do not show the diurnal mood fluctuation common to depression
(4) experience dysphoria first, followed by anxiety symptoms

285. Characteristic features of panic disorder include

(1) episodic, recurrent course
(2) signs reminiscent of myocardial infarction or hyperthyroidism
(3) anticipatory helplessness
(4) occurrence during severe stress

DIRECTIONS: Each group of questions below consists of lettered headings followed by a set of numbered items. For each numbered item select the one lettered heading with which it is most closely associated. Each lettered heading may be used once, more than once, or not at all.

Questions 286–288

Match the following.

(A) Agoraphobia
(B) Social phobia
(C) Simple phobia
(D) Both simple and social phobia
(E) None of the above

286. Generally elicited by a circumscribed stimulus

287. Characterized by marked fear and avoidance of being alone or in public places, which leads to increased limitations on normal activity

288. Characterized by persistent, irrational fear of humiliation or embarrassment

Questions 289–293

Match the following.

(A) Somatization disorder
(B) Obsessive compulsive disorder
(C) Psychogenic fugue
(D) Body dysmorphic disorder
(E) Posttraumatic stress disorder

289. After watching her house burn down, a 32-year-old woman has recurrent dreams about the event

290. A 20-year-old college student is very upset because his nose looks crooked, though to others it appears normal

291. A nun is found in a distant city, working in a cabaret, and unable to remember her previous life

292. A 35-year-old mother is anxious and upset by her inability to stop persistent impulses to stab her newborn child

293. A college student has a 3-year history of episodes of amnesia and blindness, as well as multiple chest and gastrointestinal symptoms, for which no organic cause can be discovered

Anxiety, Somatoform, and Dissociative Disorders

Answers

266. The answer is C. *(American Psychiatric Association, ed 3-R. pp 235–237.)* Panic disorder has an average age of onset in the twenties. It is found equally in males and females, though some studies suggest a slightly higher rate in the latter. When associated with agoraphobia, it is nearly twice as common in females. There is a clear familial trend, but there is controversy as to whether this is predominantly due to genetic or environmental influence. Both anxiolytic agents and antidepressants are often successful in the treatment of patients with this disorder. Effective treatment rarely requires initial hospitalization.

267. The answer is B. *(American Psychiatric Association, ed 3-R. pp 240–241.)* Panic disorder with agoraphobia is much more common than panic disorder without agoraphobia. However, occasionally patients will present with agoraphobia without a history or presence of panic disorder. In this condition the patient experiences the same fears of being in situations from which escape would be difficult, or in which help might not be available in the event that symptoms should develop. Commonly feared symptoms include becoming dizzy, loss of bladder or bowel control, and vomiting. It is unclear as to whether agoraphobia is always a variant of panic disorder.

268. The answer is D. *(American Psychiatric Association, ed 3-R. pp 269–270.)* In adults, the number of personalities in any one case of multiple personality disorder varies from two to over one hundred. Approximately half of recently reported cases have ten personalities or less. At least two of the personalities, at some time and recurrently, take full control of the person's behavior. The disorder commonly has its onset in childhood, though often it is not diagnosed until much later in life. Studies of patients with this disorder consistently reveal a high percentage who have been subjected to sexual or physical abuse in childhood.

269. The answer is A. *(American Psychiatric Association, ed 3-R. pp 251–253.)* According to the criteria of *DSM III-R*, for a diagnosis of generalized anxiety disorder there must be symptoms of unrealistic or excessive anxiety about two or more life circumstances for 6 months or longer. The spectrum of symptoms includes many signs of motor tension, autonomic hyperactivity, vigilance, and scanning. The onset is most commonly in young adulthood, the course is often chronic, and the disorder occurs with equal frequency in males and females. Often there are mild depressive symptoms, and the disorder sometimes seems to follow a major depressive episode.

270.   The answer is C. *(American Psychiatric Association, ed 3-R, pp 245-247.)* Typically patients with obsessive compulsive disorder experience their symptoms as irrational, intrusive, and irresistible. They are aware that the problem is coming from their own mind and can usually acknowledge that the belief behind their action is unfounded or unreasonable. This is in contrast to the unshakable beliefs associated with delusions. When patients with this disorder attempt to stop compulsive behavior, tension and anxiety mount to the point where it is impossible to do so. Anxiety is therefore relieved by performing a compulsion.

271.   The answer is A. *(Kaplan, ed 5, pp 1198-1199.)* Episodes of hyperventilation are associated with rapid, shallow breathing; fear or panic; and frightening physical sensations. The hyperventilation induces a respiratory alkalosis through a loss of carbon dioxide. The attempt by the body to buffer this and maintain pH produces a drop in serum calcium (which can induce tetany) and also reflex vasoconstriction that affects the skin and central nervous system. Hyperventilation syndrome is often associated with the anxiety disorders, especially panic disorder. One can usually reproduce the patient's symptoms by experimental hyperventilation or by administering an infusion of sodium lactate.

272.   The answer is B. *(Kaplan, ed 5, p 956.)* Sleep panic may occur in up to 70 percent of patients with panic disorder. The typical history is of sudden awakening from sleep with panic symptoms similar to those occurring during episodes of daytime panic. One does not see reduced REM latency in panic disorder, and sleep panic occurs during stage 2 or stage 3 sleep. It is not associated with REM sleep or with dreaming. Sleep deprivation is commonly associated with a worsening of anxiety conditions.

273.   The answer is C. *(Talbott, pp 569-579.)* Multiple personality is a very complex and chronic form of dissociative disorder consisting of the existence within the individual of two or more personalities, each of which may be dominant at a given moment and therefore may determine behavior. It is reported that 75 to 90 percent of such patients are female, and nearly all have a history of childhood abuse (physical, emotional, or sexual). The condition has its onset in childhood, usually before the age of nine. These patients very commonly have multiple psychiatric symptoms and other diagnoses, such as anxiety, depression, and borderline personality disorder.

274.   The answer is B. *(American Psychiatric Association, Treatments, pp 2046-2047.)* The antipsychotic drugs are normally not used in anxiety disorders

One exception would be a prepsychotic state with terror and anxiety that is unresponsive to benzodiazepines. Such patients may respond to low doses of neuroleptic medication. If a true psychotic process is beginning, more traditional treatment with antipsychotic drugs is in order.

275. The answer is E. (*American Psychiatric Association, Treatments, p 2047.*) Buspirone has a chemical structure different from that of benzodiazepines and has a potency on a per-milligram basis that is equivalent to that of diazepam. It takes 1 to 2 weeks for the antianxiety effects to appear, so that it is not useful for anxiety conditions that require acute intervention. Buspirone is less sedating than the benzodiazepines and appears to have less potential for abuse.

276. The answer is E. (*Kaplan, ed 5. p 968.*) Pheochromocytoma is a vascular tumor that produces catecholamines. Patients with this tumor can experience panic similar to that seen in patients with panic disorder. The diagnosis is suggested when there is a hypertensive response to smoking or malignant hypertensive episodes, crushing abdominal or back pain, or profuse sweating in the chest and back regions. Patients with anxiety disorders, including panic disorder, usually are hyperactive when anxious. Patients with pheochromocytoma characteristically want to stay very still during an episode of catecholamine release. The diagnosis can be confirmed by 24-h urine studies.

277. The answer is B. (*Kaplan, ed 5. p 1037.*) Dissociative (hysterical) amnesia may occur following head injury, either alone or in combination with postconcussional amnesia. Typically the retrograde amnesia following concussion does not extend beyond 1 week, and the recovery of memories occurs slowly and in a spotty fashion. In contrast, the recovery from hysterical amnesia is usually sudden, dramatic, and complete. Hypnosis may be helpful as a diagnostic tool. If memories are restored during a hypnotic trance, it is likely that dissociative mechanisms are at least partially responsible for the amnesia.

278. The answer is C. (*Kaplan, ed 5. p 1017.*) Hypochondriasis is defined by *DSM III-R* as a condition in which there is a persistent fear or belief, despite medical reassurance, that one has a physical illness. The belief is not of delusional proportions, and the patient's symptoms are not those of panic attacks. By definition the condition must persist for 6 months in order to make this diagnosis. It is estimated that from 3 to 14 percent of patients seen in a general medical practice may suffer from hypochondriasis.

279. The answer is C. (*Kaplan, ed 5. pp 1038–1043.*) The phenomenon of an occasional isolated depersonalization experience is quite common and occurs in both adults and children. To meet the diagnostic criteria for depersonalization disorder, as defined by *DSM III-R*, the experiences must be persistent and severe enough to cause distress, and reality testing must remain intact. In the majority of patients, symptoms appear suddenly, usually between the ages of 15 and 30. Since depersonalization can occur as a result of disturbed brain function, careful evaluation is necessary to rule out such diagnoses as brain tumor or temporal lobe epilepsy.

280. The answer is A (1, 2, 3). *(American Psychiatric Association, ed 3-R, pp 235–237. Michels, vol 1, chap 33, p 4.)* As a consequence of panic disorder, patients develop anticipatory anxiety (or generalized anxiety) apparently because they are fearful of the next anxiety attack. Frequently it is difficult for patients later to recall whether the generalized anxiety or the panic attack began first. Agoraphobia, the fear of open or crowded places, may develop as a consequence of panic attacks. Similarly, depression is not uncommon in such patients. Psychosis, however, is not associated with this disorder, even though the fear of losing one's mind, or "going crazy," is common.

281. The answer is E (all). *(American Psychiatric Association, ed 3-R, p 237.)* The differential diagnosis of panic disorder includes several physical conditions. These include disorders such as pheochromocytoma, hyperthyroidism, and hypoglycemia. Also, withdrawal from substances such as barbiturates, and intoxication with substances such as caffeine and amphetamine, can induce panic attacks.

282. The answer is A (1, 2, 3). *(Talbott, p 448.)* The locus ceruleus, located in the pons, is involved in a prominent hypothesis for the etiology of panic attacks. The hypothesis is supported by the observation that electrical stimulation of this area, or its stimulation by drugs such as yohimbine, is associated with an anxiety response. Drugs capable of blocking panic attacks, such as the tricyclic antidepressants, have been shown to curtail locus ceruleus firing. Infusions of sodium lactate induce anxiety in patients with panic disorder, but less frequently or not at all in normal controls.

283. The answer is E (all). *(American Psychiatric Association, ed 3-R, pp 274–275.)* In psychogenic amnesia there is a sudden inability to recall important personal information. During such an amnestic period the patient may exhibit perplexity, disorientation, and purposeless wandering. When the amnesia is for the past, the patient is usually aware of the disturbance of recall. In alcoholic amnestic disorder, events can be recalled immediately after they occur, but not after a few minutes. This is not seen in psychogenic amnesia. Also, the patient commonly displays blunted affect, confabulation, and a lack of awareness of the short-term memory impairment.

284. The answer is B (1, 3). *(Talbott, pp 453–454.)* The differentiation of anxiety from depression can be very difficult because anxious patients can be depressed and depressed patients can be quite anxious. Patients with generalized anxiety disorder or panic disorder generally do not show the full range of vegetative symptoms seen in a depressive episode. They may have difficulty falling asleep, but usually do not show early morning awakening, loss of appetite, loss of the ability to concentrate, or diurnal mood fluctuation. Anxious patients also do not show an equivalent loss of the capacity to enjoy things. Also, they generally give a history of having anxiety symptoms first, followed by the gradual development of dysphoric symptoms. Depressed patients usually give a history of feeling dysphoria first, with anxiety symptoms coming later. Tricyclic antidepressants are commonly used in the treatment of both panic disorder and depression.

285. The answer is A (1, 2, 3). *(Kaplan, ed 5. pp 953–959, 967–969.)* Panic disorder is a recurrent disorder characterized by acute panic anxiety and feelings of helplessness and fear preceding the panic attack. Affected persons often do remarkably well during times of severe life stress, and exertion is not known to bring about an attack. Symptoms and signs can include tremor, sweating, hyperreflexia, tachycardia, dyspnea, palpitations, and hyperventilation. As a consequence, the differential diagnosis of patients presenting with an apparent panic attack should include other disorders—such as angina, myocardial infarction, hyperthyroidism, and pheochromocytoma—also associated with these common constitutional symptoms.

286-288.   The answers are: 286-D, 287-A, 288-B. *(American Psychiatric Association, ed 3-R. pp 241–245. Michels, vol 1, chap 33, pp 6–7.)* Phobic disorders, a subclassification of anxiety disorders, include agoraphobia and simple and social phobias. They are all characterized by overwhelming, persistent, and irrational fears that result in the overpowering need to avoid the object or situation generating the dread. Agoraphobia is the marked fear and avoidance of being alone or in public places where rapid exit would be difficult. As the phobia progresses, avoidance of the stimulus dominates the person's life. Social phobia is characterized by avoidance of situations in which one is exposed to scrutiny by others and a fear of being humiliated or embarrassed by one's actions. Simple phobias are triggered by objects—often animals or insects—heights, or closed spaces. A large variety of objects are associated with simple phobias. Both social and simple phobias generally involve a circumscribed stimulus that elicits the phobic response.

289-293.   The answers are: 289-E, 290-D, 291-C, 292-B, 293-A. *(American Psychiatric Association, ed 3-R. pp 245–251, 255–256, 261–264, 272–273.)* One of the characteristic features of posttraumatic stress disorder is the occurrence of repeated dreams or recollections of the major stress event. The disturbance must persist for more than 1 month for the diagnosis to be made.

In body dysmorphic disorder, a person of normal appearance is preoccupied with some imagined insignificant physical anomaly. The belief is not of delusional intensity, for if it were it would be diagnosed as a delusional disorder. The diagnosis also specifically excludes both anorexia nervosa, wherein thin patients see themselves as obese, and transsexualism.

In psychogenic fugue, the predominant disturbance is sudden, unexpected travel, with inability to recall one's past. There is a partial or complete assumption of a new identity, often one that is more uninhibited.

Patients with obsessive compulsive disorder have persistent thoughts, impulses, or compulsions that are very stressful and that they are unable to stop by act of will. These are experienced as intrusive, senseless products of one's own mind. They are the source of much distress and interference.

In somatization disorder, a patient without evidence of organic pathology has at least 13 physical symptoms from a list that includes gastrointestinal, cardiopulmonary, sexual, conversion or pseudoneurologic, and pain symptoms. The condition begins before age 30 and usually has a chronic though fluctuating course. It is most commonly diagnosed in females.

Personality Disorders, Human Sexuality, and Miscellaneous Syndromes

DIRECTIONS: Each question below contains five suggested responses. Select the one best response to each question.

294. The differential diagnosis of obsessive compulsive personality disorder includes all the following conditions EXCEPT

(A) depression
(B) anxiety disorders
(C) phobias
(D) schizophrenia
(E) impulse disorders

295. All the following medical or psychiatric conditions are commonly associated with male erectile disorder EXCEPT

(A) diabetes mellitus
(B) manic disorder
(C) multiple sclerosis
(D) prostatectomy
(E) heroin addiction

296. All the following are associated with narcissistic personality disorder EXCEPT

(A) intense empathy
(B) fantasies of glory
(C) entitlement
(D) exploitative behavior
(E) grandiose self-importance

297. All the following statements concerning persons with avoidant personality disorder are true EXCEPT

(A) they usually appear calm during psychiatric interviews
(B) they very much want affection and are eager to please
(C) they require uncritical acceptance before entering into a relationship
(D) in their work, they usually are on the periphery of responsibility
(E) they are hypersensitive to rejection and misinterpret social interactions

298. All the following are true statements about nocturnal penile tumescence (erection) EXCEPT

(A) it typically occurs during REM sleep
(B) it is commonly measured to assist the differential diagnosis of organic versus functional impotence
(C) its presence rules out an organic basis for male erectile disorder
(D) it is commonly combined with measurement of penile rigidity
(E) it may be affected by depression

299. The most common finding in patients with factitious disorder is

(A) an associated major mental disorder
(B) an aggressive, assertive personality style
(C) frequent signing out of hospitals
(D) self-administered injections or self-medication
(E) lack of medical training

300. The diagnosis of adjustment disorder is limited to those patients who have a

(A) specific psychiatric disorder exacerbated by stress
(B) maladaptive reaction to a single, overwhelming life stress
(C) maladaptive reaction that ceases promptly after the precipitating stress has passed
(D) maladaptive dysfunctional reaction markedly out of proportion to the severity of the precipitating stress
(E) reactive disturbance of emotion but no disturbance of conduct

301. Phobias would be LEAST likely to occur in conjunction with or as manifestations of which of the following disorders?

(A) Schizophrenia
(B) Depersonalization states
(C) Sociopathy
(D) Obsessive states
(E) Anorexia nervosa

302. The capacity for female orgasm is commonly interfered with in all the following medical illnesses or treatments EXCEPT

(A) use of monoamine oxidase inhibitors
(B) use of benzodiazepines
(C) primary hyperprolactinemia
(D) diabetes mellitus
(E) hypothyroidism

303. All the following are true statements about transvestic fetishism EXCEPT

(A) it occurs in males who are homosexual
(B) there are sexual urges and arousing fantasies associated with cross-dressing
(C) masturbation is often associated with fantasies of sexual attractiveness while dressed as a woman
(D) the disorder typically begins in childhood or adolescence
(E) there is no desire for sex-reassignment surgery

304. Children who go on to develop antisocial personality disorder in adulthood would be LEAST likely to

(A) engage in thievery
(B) attempt suicide
(C) be truant
(D) stay out late
(E) run away

305. A pouting and demanding 25-year-old woman begins psychotherapy stating she is both desperate and bored. She recounts a 5- or 6-year history of short episodic bursts of anxiety and depression, several theatrical suicidal gestures, impulsive and self-defeating behavior, and sexual promiscuity. She wonders if she might be a lesbian, though most of her sexual experiences have been with men. She has abruptly terminated two previous attempts at psychotherapy when she became enraged at the therapist's unwillingness to prescribe anxiolytic medication. The mental status examination shows her reality testing to be intact, and no diagnosis is apparent on axis I. Which of the following is the most likely axis II diagnosis?

(A) Passive aggressive personality disorder
(B) Histrionic personality disorder
(C) Antisocial personality disorder
(D) Borderline personality disorder
(E) Schizotypal personality disorder

306. All the following statements describe Ganser's syndrome EXCEPT that

(A) it may be a subtype of malingering
(B) it was first described in criminals awaiting trial for serious offenses
(C) it can be mistaken for dementia
(D) affected persons' responses are unrelated to questions asked them
(E) it is considered to be a disorder of both thought and speech

307. All the following are characteristics of multiple personality disorder (MPD) EXCEPT that

(A) observers are usually unaware of personality changes
(B) MPD is considered a dissociative disorder in *DSM III-R*
(C) afflicted persons find objects in their possession they cannot account for
(D) hypnosis may facilitate diagnosis
(E) the disorder is frequently not recognized

Questions 308–310

A 33-year-old, married, male patient comes for consultation because of chronic anxiety. He states his marriage is very happy and he gives a sexual history that includes daily and satisfying sexual intercourse with his wife. He also masturbates three to four times weekly. He states that his sexual drive has been high ever since he was a teen-ager. His sexual fantasies are predominantly heterosexual, but there are occasional homosexual fantasies while masturbating. On several occasions as an adult, while traveling alone, he has had both heterosexual and homosexual experiences, which are remembered as having been pleasurable. While describing some transient guilt about "stepping out" on his wife, he is not anxious or troubled about his sexuality and does not consider it to be a problem.

308. On the basis of the patient's sexual history, one could reasonably infer a diagnosis of

(A) schizotypal personality disorder
(B) antisocial personality disorder
(C) narcissistic personality disorder
(D) borderline personality disorder
(E) none of the above

309. Which of the following statements is most likely to be true about the patient's masturbation and frequency of total sexual outlet?

(A) The patient has a higher-than-average sexual drive, but it is within the range of normal
(B) Regular masturbation in a married man, for whom intercourse is available, is pathologic
(C) The patient is probably hypomanic
(D) The regularity of his masturbation makes it very probable that he has falsely characterized sexuality with his wife as satisfying
(E) The patient is probably psychotic

310. Which of the following statements is most likely to be true about the history of occasional homosexual fantasies and several adult homosexual experiences?

(A) The patient is almost certainly a repressed homosexual
(B) The absence of anxiety or concern about his sexuality suggests psychopathology
(C) He may be bisexual, but there is nothing in the history to suggest sexual psychopathology
(D) There is a need for conjoint marital therapy
(E) The patient likely has a disturbance of core gender identity

DIRECTIONS: Each question below contains four suggested responses of which **one or more** is correct. Select

A	if	**1, 2, and 3**	are correct
B	if	**1 and 3**	are correct
C	if	**2 and 4**	are correct
D	if	**4**	is correct
E	if	**1, 2, 3, and 4**	are correct

311. Advantages of multidimensional self-rated instruments used to assess personality include which of the following?

(1) They provide useful supplementary information
(2) They assist in making diagnostic and treatment decisions
(3) They are relatively cost-effective
(4) They diminish the possibility of inter-rater bias

312. Schizoid personality disorder is differentiated from schizotypal personality disorder by

(1) an absence of close relationships and friends
(2) constricted affect
(3) avoidance of social situations
(4) an absence of oddities of behavior, perception, and speech

313. Empirically based psychometric instruments used to assess personality disorders include which of the following?

(1) Minnesota Multiphasic Personality Inventory (MMPI)
(2) Thematic Apperception Test (TAT)
(3) Clinical Analysis Questionnaire (CAQ)
(4) Profile of Mood State (POMS)

314. The circumplex model is useful in making the diagnosis of which of the following conditions?

(1) Schizophrenia
(2) Anxiety disorders
(3) Somatoform disorders
(4) Personality disorders

315. Medical complications commonly found in bulimia nervosa include

(1) hypokalemic alkalosis
(2) parotid gland enlargement
(3) cardiac arrhythmias or failure
(4) gastric dilatation

316. True statements concerning personality disorders include that

(1) personality disorders are relatively superficial and respond well to therapy
(2) personality disorders cause impairment in adaptive functioning or subjective distress
(3) persons with personality disorders can have periods of remission up to a year
(4) personality disorders are evident by adolescence or earlier

SUMMARY OF DIRECTIONS

A	B	C	D	E
1, 2, 3	1, 3	2, 4	4	All are
only	only	only	only	correct

Questions 317–319

A 17-year-old high-school senior, who is 168 cm (66 in) tall and weighs 31.8 kg (70 lb), is admitted to the hospital. She talks a great deal about fears of "losing control" and becoming fat. She diets rigorously and exercises faithfully, and, though emaciated in appearance, she insists that her cheeks, abdomen, hips, and thighs are too heavy. She is unconcerned that her menstrual periods have ceased. The clinical staff notes that, though busy about the kitchen on her ward, she orders dietary food, spreads it about her plate, and eats little. Her parents are concerned about her weight but are not sure she should be hospitalized.

317. Important symptoms and signs associated with this condition include

(1) striving for thinness
(2) altered body image
(3) amenorrhea
(4) behavioral problems at home

318. Clinical and laboratory examination of the girl described would be likely to reveal

(1) bradycardia
(2) elevated serum carotene concentration
(3) hypotension and hypothermia
(4) leukopenia

319. The girl described is likely to

(1) ignore concerns about dying
(2) display a strong wish to remain passively dependent
(3) have obsessional traits
(4) have an underlying depression

320. According to the criteria of *DSM III-R*, personality disorders are

(1) coded on axis II
(2) not diagnosed in the presence of major mental illness
(3) recognizable by adolescence or early adult life
(4) not associated with impairment of social and vocational functioning

321. Anorexia nervosa is characterized by which of the following?

(1) An intense fear of obesity
(2) Distorted body image—"feeling fat" even when emaciated
(3) Refusal to maintain weight over minimum normal weight
(4) Weight loss of at least 35 percent of original body weight

322. Characteristics of people who have paranoid personality disorder include

(1) overconcern with hidden motives and special meanings
(2) preoccupation with helping the weak and powerless
(3) extreme reluctance to enter into psychotherapy
(4) predisposition to develop schizophrenia

323. Persons with antisocial personality disorder typically do which of the following?

(1) Convey an impression of intelligence to psychiatric examiners
(2) Explain their behavior away with an appropriate expression of feeling
(3) "Burn out" (i.e., remit) by mid-adulthood
(4) Respond to a brief course of limit-setting psychotherapy

DIRECTIONS: Each group of questions below consists of four lettered headings followed by a set of numbered items. For each numbered item select

A	if the item is associated with	(A) only
B	if the item is associated with	(B) only
C	if the item is associated with	both (A) and (B)
D	if the item is associated with	neither (A) nor (B)

Each lettered heading may be used once, more than once, or not at all.

Questions 324–328

(A) Schizoid personality disorder
(B) Avoidant personality disorder
(C) Both
(D) Neither

324. Hypersensitivity to rejection

325. Few personal attachments

326. Absence of warm, tender feelings for others

327. Common presence of eccentricities of speech and behavior

328. Low self-esteem

Questions 329–330

(A) Transsexualism
(B) Gender identity disorder of adolescence or adulthood, nontranssexual type (GIDAANT)
(C) Both
(D) Neither

329. Persistent discomfort and sense of inappropriateness about one's assigned sex

330. Cross-dressing for the purpose of sexual excitement

Personality Disorders, Human Sexuality, and Miscellaneous Syndromes

Answers

294. The answer is E. *(Kaplan, ed 5. pp 997-998.)* Obsessive compulsive personality features can be associated with several psychiatric disorders. They can occur in depressive syndromes as well as in phobic states. An increase in obsessional thinking and compulsive behavior may herald a schizophrenic breakdown. Obsessive compulsive people typically are cautious, controlled, and anxious, in contrast to people who have impulse disorders.

295. The answer is B. *(Kaplan, ed 5. pp 1051-1052.)* It is estimated that 20 to 50 percent of males with erectile disorder (impotence) have an organic basis to their problem. This is usually secondary to surgery or because of neurologic or vascular problems associated with medical illness. Impotence is also common secondary to either prescribed drugs (e.g., antihypertensives, lithium, monoamine oxidase inhibitors) or abused drugs (e.g., cocaine, heroin, morphine, alcohol). Impotence is not particularly associated with manic episodes, wherein patients are often hypersexual in their behavior.

296. The answer is A. *(Talbott, pp 632-633.)* All the listed characteristics are found in narcissistic personality disorder except empathy. Patients with this disorder are notable for their lack of empathy and consideration for the feelings of others. This is associated with a grandiose sense of self-importance and a sense of entitlement. As a result their relationships tend to be self-centered and shallow.

297. The answer is A. *(Kaplan, ed 5. p 1380.)* Persons with an avoidant personality disorder are anxious, often strikingly so, during psychiatric interviews. They typically are eager to please yet are oversensitive to perceived rejection. Despite low self-esteem and avoidance of risk, these persons desire almost desperately to be in the social and occupational mainstream. Usually, however, their relationships are distorted by their exquisite sensitivity to rejection, and they gravitate toward work roles far from the spotlight. Alliance with a therapist and assertiveness training may be quite helpful to persons who have avoidant personality disorder.

298. The answer is C. *(Kaplan, ed 5. pp 1051-1053.)* The monitoring of nocturnal penile tumescence (NPT) is a common procedure to help differentiate organic from functional impotence. In 85 to 90 percent of cases, the presence of erections that normally accompany REM sleep will rule out a physical basis for the problem. However, men with conditions such as hyperprolactinemia or subtle vascular disorders may have erections during their REM sleep. Conversely, studies may show decreased tumescence in the absence of organic disorder, for example in some males with depression. NPT studies are not usually necessary if the patient reports spontaneous erections, morning erections, or good erections with masturbation.

299. The answer is D. *(Michels, vol 1, chap 35, pp 16-19.)* Patients with factitious disorders are often medical professionals or people closely associated with and knowledgeable about hospitals. Self-administered injections or ingestions of medication or foreign material (e.g., insulin, contaminants producing infection, or unacknowledged misuse of prescribed medication) are typical modes of simulating illness. These people are often passive and immature and create much controversy and anxiety in personnel who are treating them. When these patients are confronted with the diagnosis of factitious disorder, their abnormal behavior is best interpreted to them as their cry for help. Suicide attempts and signing out of hospitals are infrequent even after confrontation. These patients are not sociopathic, nor do they usually manifest psychiatric disorders.

300. The answer is D. *(Kaplan, ed 5. pp 1141-1142.)* Adjustment disorders are characterized by temporary maladaptive behavior or symptom patterns that are markedly out of proportion to the precipitating stress or stresses. Onset of the disorder may not be coincident with occurrence of the precipitating stressful event, and symptoms may continue well beyond the cessation of the stress. Disturbances of both emotion and conduct may occur in association with adjustment disorders. This diagnosis, however, should not be made when other, specific psychiatric disorders are clearly present.

301. The answer is C. *(Kaplan, ed 5. pp 980-982.)* Phobias can exist in association with schizophrenic decompensation and may be the initial manifestation of obsessions. People who have anorexia nervosa have phobic fears of losing control of their eating habits and becoming fat. Phobic attacks can be a major aspect in depersonalization states, as exemplified by the phobic anxiety-depersonalization syndrome. Phobias are not likely to be associated with sociopathic personality disorders.

302. The answer is B. *(Kaplan, ed 5. p 1053.)* There are a number of medical illnesses and treatments that are associated with reduced capacity for female orgasm. Diabetes mellitus, hypothyroidism, and primary hyperprolactinemia are commonly implicated. A number of drugs, such as antihypertensives and some antidepressants, may similarly interfere. Benzodiazepines do not commonly inhibit either male erectile function or the capacity for f€ ale orgasm.

303. The answer is A. *(American Psychiatric Association, ed 3-R, pp 288-289.)* Transvestic fetishism is a condition that occurs in heterosexual males who experience recurrent and intensely sexually exciting urges involving cross-dressing. While cross-dressed, there is often masturbation with fantasies of sexual attractiveness while dressed as a woman. Wearing an article of clothing, or dressing as a woman, can also be sexually exciting while having intercourse. The condition typically begins in childhood or early adolescence. Males with this disorder consider themselves to be male and have no desire for sex-reassignment surgery.

304. The answer is B. *(Kaplan, ed 5. pp 1373-1376.)* Suicide attempts are rare in children who develop antisocial personality disorder in adulthood. These children seem to act out their problems in ways other than self-destruction. Theft, incorrigibility, truancy, running away, bad companions, staying out late, and physical aggression all are associated commonly with children who become antisocial adults.

305. The answer is D. *(American Psychiatric Association, ed 3-R, pp 346-347.)* The history and findings are classic for the diagnosis of borderline personality disorder. These patients present with the history of a pervasive instability of mood, relationships, and self-image beginning by early adulthood. Their behavior is often impulsive and self-damaging, their sexuality is chaotic, sexual orientation may be uncertain, and anger is intense and often acted out. Recurrent suicidal gestures or behavior is common. The shifts of mood and anxiety are usually brief, lasting from a few hours to a few days. Patients often describe chronic feelings of boredom and emptiness.

306. The answer is D. *(Kaplan, ed 5. p 1139.)* The major characteristic of Ganser's syndrome is that affected persons respond to questions in an appropriate form—as if they understood the questions—but at the same time give absolutely incorrect answers. Thus, rather than being unrelated to the questions asked, these responses may be thought to parallel the correct responses; in fact, Ganser's syndrome may be mistaken for dementia, until the parallelism of these responses is discerned. The syndrome, which is considered to be a disorder of thought and speech, may be a subtype of malingering. It was first described in prison inmates, most of whom were awaiting trial for murder.

307. The answer is A. *(American Psychiatric Association, ed 3-R, pp 269-272. Michels, vol 1, chap 39, pp 8-10.)* Descriptions of multiple personalities in the psychiatric literature are often colorful and dramatic, yet many psychiatrists remain skeptical about the occurrence of this disorder. Multiple personality disorder is currently classified in *DSM III-R* as a type of dissociative disorder. One factor that may lead clinicians to be skeptical about the occurrence of the disorder is that it is frequently not recognized. The afflicted person takes on other personalities of which the "host" personality is unaware. As a result the afflicted person may be told of events or behavior that he or she cannot remember. Objects may be found in the person's possession that cannot be accounted for. The diagnosis may be facilitated by hypnosis and might be considered if marked changes in behavior are noted by others.

308–310.   The answers are: 308–E, 309–A, 310–C. *(Kaplan, ed 5. pp 1045–1061, 1086–1094. Talbott, pp 600–601.)* There is nothing in the patient's history to suggest the presence of a personality disorder. The hallmark of a personality disorder is the presence of a constellation of behaviors or traits that cause significant impairment in social or occupational functioning, or subjective distress. There is no history of such distress or dysfunction. While some persons in our society might object to his sexual behavior on moral grounds, such judgments are not a part of the diagnostic process.

The patient gives a history of having an average of 9 to 11 orgasms per week and describes a high sexual drive since his teens. While this frequency is higher than that found in most males in their early thirties, it is neither outside the range of normalcy nor in and of itself pathologic. Similarly, the occurrence of masturbation in married men is not particularly unusual and in and of itself does not suggest a sexual disorder or marital problems. It may be due to a higher desire level than can be satisfied with his partner, it may be a relief for sexual impulses that cannot be otherwise satisfied, or it may simply be an enjoyed alternative release. Since masturbation is sometimes motivated by a desire to reduce anxiety rather than to satisfy sexual drive, it may also be related to his general anxiety. Patients who are manic or hypomanic often have increased sexual drive and frequency of release, but this tends to be episodic rather than consistent and lifelong.

Sexual behavior and fantasies range on a continuum from exclusively heterosexual to exclusively homosexual. There are many men who are predominantly heterosexual but who have engaged in homosexual behavior or have occasional homosexual fantasies, and there are many predominantly homosexual men with capacity for heterosexual arousal. The presence of homosexual desire or behavior is not considered, according to the diagnostic definitions of the American Psychiatric Association, to constitute a sexual disorder. While further therapeutic inquiry may uncover sexual conflict or marital disorder, the current history does not necessarily suggest that will be the case.

311.   The answer is E (all). *(Michels, vol 1, chap 15, p 11.)* The advantages of multidimensional self-reported instruments, like the MMPI, are that they provide useful supplemental information for the clinician and assist in decisions of diagnosis and treatment. They are cost-effective and can now be done on computer monitors, thereby greatly diminishing inter-rater bias.

312.   The answer is D (4). *(American Psychiatric Association, ed 3-R, pp 339-342.)* In schizotypal personality disorder there are not only deficits in interpersonal relatedness, but peculiarities of ideation, appearance, and behavior beginning by early adulthood. These peculiarities are not a part of the diagnosis of schizoid personality disorder. In both conditions there may be constricted affect, but in schizotypal personality disorder the affect may also be quite inappropriate. People with either disorder tend not to have close relationships and to be uncomfortable in social situations.

313.   The answer is B (1, 3). *(Michels, vol 1, chap 15, pp 5-6.)* The MMPI and CAQ are empirically based tests of personality. They are scored by matching the subject's responses to those of people with known disorders or traits. The TAT is a projective test in which the subject interprets a series of pictures. The POMS assesses a subject's current mood state via rating how the subject feels in regard to mood adjectives.

314.   The answer is D (4). *(Michels, vol 1, chap 15, pp 8-11.)* The circumplex model is a two-dimensional circular ordering of ideas or concepts based on their similarities. For over 30 years it has been used to describe the structure of personality traits. Theoretically, traits close in proximity within the circle are similar, whereas those opposite one another represent bipolarities.

315.   The answer is E (all). *(Talbott, p 761.)* Patients with bulimia nervosa engage in self-induced vomiting or use of laxatives or diuretics. They are susceptible to the development of hypokalemic alkalosis and other electrolyte disturbances. These disturbances may induce cardiac arrhythmia, and this can lead to cardiac arrest. Parotid gland enlargement, with elevated serum amylase levels, is common in patients who binge and vomit. Gastric dilatation is a rare complication in patients who binge and should be considered an emergency condition.

316.   The answer is C (2, 4). *(Kaplan, ed 5, pp 1352-1354.)* DSM III-R describes personality disorders as deeply ingrained, inflexible, maladaptive patterns of relating to, perceiving, and thinking about the environment and oneself that result in impairment in adaptive functioning or subjective distress. They are pervasive personality traits and are generally recognized by the time of adolescence or earlier and continue throughout most of adult life.

317-319.   The answers are: 317-A (1, 2, 3), 318-E (all), 319-A (1, 2, 3). *(Kaplan, ed 5, pp 1858-1860.)* Amenorrhea, an altered body image, and an energetic striving for thinness compose the "classic triad" of symptoms and signs of persons who have anorexia nervosa. The often profound cachexia of these persons is usually accompanied by flagrantly distorted ideation about their bodies and by earnest efforts, such as exercising and dieting, to lose what they consider excess weight. In approximately half of all affected girls and women, loss of menstruation occurs before loss of weight. Fear of losing control, lack of concern about loss of menses, constipation, and the classic "good girl" description are other aspects of anorexia nervosa. Among the clinical and laboratory features of anorexia nervosa are bradycardia, leukopenia, hypotension, hypothermia, and elevated serum levels of carotene. Leukopenia, along with malnutrition, may lead to potentially fatal infections. Despite considerable inanition, persons who have this disorder tend to be bright, alert, energetic, and resourceful; in addition, most remain unaware of the life-threatening potential of their disrupted eating habits. Obsessional traits commonly are associated with anorexia nervosa, as is the strong wish to remain passively dependent. Although poor appetite and weight loss may accompany deep depression, underlying depression is unusual in persons affected by anorexia nervosa.

320. The answer is B (1, 3). *(American Psychiatric Association, ed 3-R, pp 335-336.)* Personality disorders represent a constellation of traits or behaviors that are characteristic of the person's recent and long-term functioning and are recognized by adolescence or early adulthood. They are often associated with very significant social and vocational impairment. Personality disorders are coded on axis II and may coexist with axis I diagnoses.

321. The answer is A (1, 2, 3). *(American Psychiatric Association, ed 3-R, pp 65-67. Kaplan, ed 5. pp 1859-1862.)* Anorexia nervosa occurs predominantly in women, particularly in adolescents and young adults. It is characterized by an intense fear of obesity, distorted body image, and progressive weight loss. The mortality has not been definitely established but is probably about 10 percent. Current criteria specify that the patient must have lost at least 25 percent of original body weight in order to warrant the diagnosis of anorexia nervosa.

322. The answer is B (1, 3). *(Kaplan, ed 5. pp 1365-1366.)* Persons with paranoid personality disorder are markedly suspicious of others. They are intensely alert to any potential disloyalty, threat, or injustice, and they are typically overconcerned with perceived hidden motives or special meanings in the behavior of others. Although they may be moralistic, self-righteous, and litigious, paranoid persons are acutely sensitive to matters of power and status and are usually contemptuous of the weak and helpless. Because of the nature of their disorder, affected persons usually are very reluctant to enter into psychotherapy. When they do enter therapy, therapists do best by maintaining a carefully professional, somewhat distant attitude. The epidemiology of paranoid personality disorder is not well established. The percentage of affected persons who go on to develop frank schizophrenia is not known.

323. The answer is B (1, 3). *(Kaplan, ed 5. pp 1373-1377.)* People who have antisocial personality disorder often are colorful, superficially charming, and manipulative. In addition, many seem quite intelligent. However, affect typically is not in proportion to behavior—that is, they tend to present bland rationalizations of their actions. Antisocial behavior most often is displayed by teenagers and young adults, with decreasing prevalence rates thereafter. However, up to one-third of persons with antisocial personality disorder become alcoholic. Treatment, which usually involves lengthy, repetitive limit-setting, often is complicated by well-meaning "rescuers" who continually extricate these people from difficulty, allowing them to return promptly to their antisocial ways.

324-328.   The answers are: 324-B, 325-C, 326-A, 327-D, 328-B. *(American Psychiatric Association, ed 3-R, pp 339-340, 351-352.)* Patients with avoidant and schizoid personality disorders share the trait of having few close personal attachments. However, while the schizoid person is emotionally cold and aloof with an absence of tender feelings for others and indifference to praise or criticism, the avoidant person is hypersensitive to rejection and desirous of affection and acceptance, but unwilling to enter into relationships for fear of rejection. Neither are characterized by eccentricities of speech or behavior, as seen in the schizotypal personality. Even though neither avoidant nor schizoid persons will have many personal relationships, the avoidant person experiences much more psychic pain than does the schizoid person. This is a key differential feature.

329-330.   The answers are: 329-C, 330-D. *(American Psychiatric Association, ed 3-R, pp 74-77, 288-289.)* Transsexualism and gender identity disorder of adolescence or adulthood, nontranssexual type (GIDAANT) share in common a persistent discomfort and sense of inappropriateness about one's assigned sex, as well as a wish to live as a member of the opposite sex. The diagnoses are restricted to persons who are pubertal or older. Transsexualism, in contrast to GIDAANT, is associated with a preoccupation, of 2 years or longer, with getting rid of one's primary and secondary sex characteristics and taking on those of the opposite sex. While cross-dressing occurs in both diagnoses, it is not primarily for the purpose of sexual excitement, as it is in transvestic fetishism.

Alcoholism and Substance Abuse

DIRECTIONS: Each question below contains five suggested responses. Select the one best response to each question.

331. In people with normal liver function, alcohol is metabolized at

(A) 0.5 ounce per hour
(B) 1 ounce per hour
(C) 5 ounces per hour
(D) 0.5 ounce per minute
(E) 1 ounce per minute

332. Another primary psychiatric illness should be seriously considered if a psychosis, precipitated by ingestion of a hallucinogen, should persist beyond

(A) 2 h
(B) 24 h
(C) 48 h
(D) 2 weeks
(E) 6 weeks

333. Signs of intoxication may appear when the blood alcohol level reaches

(A) 30 mg/dL
(B) 150 mg/dL
(C) 2 percent
(D) 5 percent
(E) 10 percent

334. All the following disturbed sexual functions are commonly found in alcoholic persons EXCEPT

(A) decreased sperm production and motility in men
(B) decreased ejaculate volume in men
(C) increased testosterone levels in men
(D) impotence
(E) menstrual irregularities in women

335. Death can occur at a serum alcohol level of

(A) 30 mg/dL
(B) 200 mg/dL
(C) 500 mg/dL
(D) 800 mg/dL
(E) 1000 mg/dL

336. True statements about probable genetic factors in the genesis of primary alcoholism include all the following EXCEPT

(A) the concordance for alcoholism is higher in monozygotic than in dizygotic twins
(B) children who have been separated from their alcoholic biologic parents early in life have markedly elevated rates of alcoholism
(C) the children of nonalcoholics adopted into the homes of alcoholics do not show elevated rates of alcoholism as adults
(D) there is an increased intensity of reaction to ethanol in the sons and daughters of alcoholic fathers
(E) alcoholism is probably a genetically influenced disorder with a rate of heritability similar to that expected for diabetes or peptic ulcer

---

Questions 337–339

A 35-year-old man stumbles into the emergency room. His pulse is 100 beats per minute, his blood pressure is 170/95 mmHg, and he is diaphoretic. He is tremulous and has difficulty relating a history. He does admit to insomnia the past two nights and thinks a curtain is a ghost in the room. He also states he has been a drinker since age 19, but has not had a drink in 4 days.

337. The most likely diagnosis is

(A) adjustment disorder
(B) atypical psychosis
(C) alcohol withdrawal delirium (delirium tremens)
(D) alcohol intoxication
(E) alcohol idiosyncratic intoxication

338. Initial drug treatment usually includes

(A) haloperidol 10 mg IM
(B) chlorpromazine 50 mg IM
(C) lithium 300 mg PO
(D) chlordiazepoxide 50 mg PO
(E) imipramine 50 mg PO

339. Appropriate follow-up treatment for this patient would include all the following EXCEPT

(A) complete history and physical examination with emphasis on hepatic, gastrointestinal, and neurologic functioning
(B) psychological assessment to determine underlying psychopathology
(C) social assessment to identify social or environmental stressors contributing to the problem
(D) referral to alcoholics anonymous (AA)
(E) fluphenazine decanoate (Prolixin), 1 mL IM, with an appointment to his local mental health clinic for follow-up

340. Which of the following drugs is a narcotic antagonist?

(A) Chlordiazepoxide
(B) Haloperidol (Haldol)
(C) Methadone (Dolophine)
(D) Phenobarbital
(E) Naloxone (Narcan)

341. All the following statements about alcoholism are true EXCEPT

(A) current classifications of alcoholic disorders are based on etiologic factors
(B) the consequences, rather than the actual amount, of drinking may be the best means for detecting alcoholism
(C) cultural background may affect the incidence of alcoholism
(D) the tendency for alcoholism to run in families is a well-established observation
(E) the reported incidence of alcoholism in women is substantially lower than in men

342. A 39-year-old man enters an emergency room complaining of anxiety and extreme sleeplessness. He is noted to be markedly tremulous, and while being examined he has a grand mal seizure. This man might be suffering from withdrawal from any of the following substances EXCEPT

(A) alcohol
(B) haloperidol (Haldol)
(C) meprobamate (Equanil and Miltown)
(D) phenobarbital
(E) diazepam (Valium)

343. True statements about withdrawal from stimulants such as cocaine and amphetamines include all the following EXCEPT

(A) it may begin insidiously while the person is still taking stimulants
(B) it may include muscular aches and pains
(C) the first 9 h to 14 days are characterized by a "crash" with intense craving, agitation, depression, and insomnia
(D) following an initial acute phase of reaction, a period of fatigue, anxiety, and anhedonia occurs, which can last up to 10 weeks
(E) the usual treatment consists of weaning the patient from the drug by giving smaller and smaller doses

344. Wernicke-Korsakoff syndrome is seen in chronic alcohol abuse and is characterized by all the following symptoms EXCEPT

(A) ataxia
(B) nystagmus and paralysis of certain ocular muscles
(C) confabulation
(D) loss of remote memory
(E) confusion

345. Delirium tremens, which can develop in persons who abstain from drinking after a prolonged period of alcohol use, is characteristically associated with all the following EXCEPT

(A) bradycardia
(B) tremor
(C) vivid visual hallucinations
(D) disorientation to time and place
(E) a course of 3 to 7 days

346. There is good evidence that marijuana smoking significantly decreases one's ability to drive an automobile for up to

(A) 1 h
(B) 2 h
(C) 4 h
(D) 8 h
(E) 24 h

347. All the following are commonly used in the emergency treatment of acute toxic reaction secondary to phencyclidine (PCP) use EXCEPT

(A) alkalinization of the urine
(B) phentolamine (Regitine) drip
(C) benzodiazepines
(D) haloperidol (Haldol)
(E) gastric lavage

348. True statements about the nature and effects of caffeine include all the following EXCEPT

(A) it often worsens the symptoms of panic disorder of agoraphobia
(B) withdrawal symptoms occur with sudden cessation of chronic use
(C) flashbacks occur with toxic reactions secondary to overdose
(D) overdose is associated with anxiety, derealization, dizziness, and tinnitus
(E) the half-life of many caffeinated substances is about 3 to 7 h

DIRECTIONS: Each question below contains four suggested responses of which **one or more** is correct. Select

A	if	**1, 2, and 3**	are correct
B	if	**1 and 3**	are correct
C	if	**2 and 4**	are correct
D	if	**4**	is correct
E	if	**1, 2, 3, and 4**	are correct

349. Symptoms suggestive of schizophrenia are seen in the use of which of the following substances?

(1) Cocaine
(2) LSD
(3) Amphetamines
(4) Mescaline

350. Intoxication with cocaine in the chronic user may be associated with

(1) paranoid psychosis
(2) hyperreflexia and seizures
(3) euphoria and pressured speech tachycardia and mydriasis

351. Diagnostic criteria for alcohol dependence include which of the following?

(1) A pattern of pathologic alcohol use
(2) Impairment in social or occupational functioning due to alcohol use
(3) A need for increased amounts of alcohol to achieve the desired effect
(4) Development of withdrawal symptoms after stopping or reducing drinking

352. The major physiologic effects of cocaine include potent

(1) local anesthetic action
(2) sympathomimetic action
(3) stimulation of the central nervous system
(4) vasodilatation, which produces hypotension

353. Drugs that can produce a psychosis whose symptoms are strikingly similar to those of paranoid schizophrenia include

(1) cocaine
(2) methylphenidate
(3) amphetamines
(4) propranolol

354. Abuse of glue and other volatile solvents can be described by which of the following statements?

(1) Glue sniffing is most common in children and teen-agers
(2) Glue sniffing leads to intoxication similar to that caused by alcohol, and amnesia for the episode may occur
(3) Inhaling volatile substances can cause irreversible damage to brain, liver, and kidneys
(4) Inhaling volatile substances can result in death by respiratory arrest

355. Intoxication with phencyclidine (PCP) is characteristically associated with

(1) vertical and horizontal nystagmus
(2) hypotension
(3) myoclonus and ataxia
(4) sedation

356. Correct statements about alcohol abuse in the United States include which of the following?

(1) It is the second most serious drug-abuse problem
(2) During the 15 years prior to 1980 the per capita consumption of alcohol increased
(3) A cause-and-effect relationship exists between the amount of alcohol consumed and the incidence of alcoholism
(4) Approximately 10 million people are alcoholic

357. The neuropsychiatric changes often associated with meperidine (Demerol) include

(1) serene detachment
(2) dysphoria and irritability
(3) cataplexy
(4) myoclonic twitches

358. The treatment of opiate addiction can be described by which of the following statements?

(1) Medication is often used in the detoxification phase of treatment
(2) Clonidine suppresses some of the opiate-withdrawal symptoms
(3) Methadone is popular in the maintenance treatment of narcotic addiction because of its ability to block the euphoric effects of narcotic drugs
(4) Narcotic antagonists are used for treating heroin overdose but not for preventing and treating narcotic addiction

359. True statements about alcohol idiosyncratic intoxication (pathologic intoxication) include which of the following?

(1) It usually begins slowly
(2) It occurs after a large alcohol intake
(3) It involves vivid recall ("flashbacks") for the period of time involved
(4) It may involve aggressive behavior toward self and others

DIRECTIONS: The group of questions below consists of lettered headings followed by a set of numbered items. For each numbered item select the one lettered heading with which it is most closely associated. Each lettered heading may be used once, more than once, or not at all.

Questions 360–363

Match the following.

(A) Tolerance
(B) Potentiation
(C) Withdrawal
(D) Dependence
(E) Addiction

360. A repertoire of behaviors that maintain drug use

361. Requirement of a larger dose of the drug to obtain the same effect

362. A physiologic state that follows cessation of or reduction in drug use

363. A syndrome of clinically significant symptoms following cessation of substance use

Alcoholism and
Substance Abuse

Answers

331. The answer is B. *(Kaplan, ed 5. pp 687-688.)* For the average healthy person, alcohol is metabolized at the rate of 1 ounce of alcoholic drink per hour. Other factors that will influence the blood alcohol level include prior drinking history, body size, and the amount of food in the stomach. There is a range in the rate at which alcohol is metabolized by the liver. The rate is determined by the activity of the enzyme alcohol dehydrogenase and varies among cultural and ethnic groups.

332. The answer is D. *(Stoudemire, p 249.)* Most cases of intoxication with a hallucinogen are over within several hours. But prolonged drug-induced psychoses may occur, especially with PCP, in which the psychosis may last 2 to 7 days. In some instances the drug appears to precipitate a latent psychotic illness, and if the psychosis persists beyond 2 weeks, this should be seriously considered.

333. The answer is A. *(Michels, vol 2, chap 35, p 3.)* Signs of intoxication may, in some people, appear with a blood alcohol level as low as 30 mg/dL. Most people become significantly uncoordinated when their blood alcohol level reaches 0.1 percent. Some research has shown task impairment to begin at blood alcohol levels of about 0.5 percent. Blood alcohol level is influenced by the amount of alcohol as well as by body weight.

334. The answer is C. *(Schuckit, ed 3. p 60.)* Sexual functioning is commonly disturbed in persons who abuse alcohol. Alcohol has a direct effect on the testes, which may contribute to the commonly encountered impotence and decreased sprerm production and motility. Ejaculate volume is often reduced, and there is decreased production of testosterone. In women, alcohol abuse can lead to menstrual irregularities as well as to adverse effects on the developing fetus.

335. The answer is D. *(Kaplan, ed 5. p 1434.)* An inexperienced drinker can show signs of intoxication at 30 mg/dL; virtually everyone is intoxicated at a level of 200 mg/dL. Unconsciousness usually occurs at a level of 500 mg/dL and death usually occurs between 600 and 800 mg/dL. Unconsciousness usually occurs before one can drink enough to die.

336. The answer is D. *(Schuckit, ed 3. pp 68-70.)* Adoption and other family studies have consistently supported the premise that alcoholism is a genetically influenced disorder. Most investigators believe that genetic factors place a person at a higher or lower level of vulnerability, with these genetic factors then interacting with environmental ones to give a final level of risk. Numerous studies have found that the sons and daughters of alcoholic fathers have a decreased intensity of reaction to ethanol. It is postulated that this may make it more difficult for one to perceive the internal feelings that would normally alert one to the fact it was time to stop drinking.

337-339. The answers are: 337-C, 338-D, 339-E. *(Kaplan, ed 5. pp 203-204, 694-695.)* Alcohol withdrawal delirium (delirium tremens) is the severest form of alcohol withdrawal. Five percent of all hospitalized alcoholics develop delirium tremens during their hospital course. Clinically, delirium tremens develops 2 to 7 days after cessation of drinking and is characterized by tachycardia, diaphoresis, hypertension, confusion, insomnia, illusions or visual hallucinations, and tremor. Delirium tremens is most common in people with at least a 5-year drinking history in which binges are common. Initial treatment usually involves chlordiazepoxide, 50 to 100 mg. Phenothiazines should not be used because of neurologic problems and probable preexisting hepatic impairment. Follow-up treatment should include a complete biopsychosocial evaluation. AA is an excellent referral resource.

340. The answer is E. *(Kaplan, ed 5. pp 656-661.)* Naloxone (Narcan) is an opiate antagonist. Such agents, which are not addictive, block the action of opiate compounds, thus curtailing their effects. Methadone (Dolophine) is a drug whose pharmacologic properties are similar to those of morphine. The chronic administration of methadone produces both tolerance and physical dependence. By inducing tolerance to opiate-like drugs, methadone is thought to block the euphoric effects of "street" narcotics, such as heroin.

341. The answer is A. *(Kaplan, ed 5. pp 686-697.)* Existing classifications of alcoholic disorders are predominantly descriptive; in most cases the etiology is obscure. The best means of detecting alcoholism is by being alert to the possibility in persons presenting with frequently occurring sequelae—physical, social, and psychological—of alcohol abuse. Cultural, ethnic, and social factors seem to affect prevalence rates of alcoholism; in some immigrant groups, the characteristic rate of alcoholism may persist for several generations in the United States, before equaling the national norm. It is well established that alcoholism tends to run in families. More men than women still are reported to be alcoholic, but this discrepancy may reflect in part the fact that women are able to "hide" their alcohol problem with less difficulty.

342.   The answer is B. *(Kaplan, ed 5. pp 666–667, 1594.)* Haloperidol (Haldol) is an antipsychotic agent of the butyrophenone class. It does not produce the classic physical dependence and withdrawal effects that are associated with alcohol and antianxiety agents, such as diazepam, meprobamate (Equanil and Miltown), and phenobarbital. As in the case described in the question, symptoms of withdrawal from these agents can include tremor, insomnia, and seizures.

343.   The answer is E. *(Schuckit, ed 3. pp 111–113.)* Withdrawal from stimulants such as cocaine and amphetamines can be insidious or more dramatic, and the phenomenon of tolerance makes it possible for withdrawal to occur while the patient is still taking the drug. Typical symptoms during the "crash" period (9 h to 14 days) include muscular aches, intense craving, intense agitation, decreased appetite, and finally depression. After a while fatigue and insomnia appear, the craving is decreased, and there is a sense of exhaustion. Following this phase, the next 1 to 10 weeks is associated with less depression and craving, but there is a recurrence of fatigue, anxiety, and anhedonia. A craving for the drug often persists for a long time. Treatment is abrupt withdrawal rather than tapering, along with supportive intervention.

344.   The answer is D. *(Schuckit, ed 3. p 82.)* Wernicke-Korsakoff syndrome is associated with chronic alcohol abuse. It results from the fact that in the presence of alcohol, thiamine is not absorbed adequately and is metabolized at a faster rate. Neurologic symptoms include ataxia, nystagmus, and paralysis of certain c muscles. As with all organic brain syndromes, the primary effect is a decrease recent memory function as opposed to remote memory. Other psychological symptoms include confusion, as well as confabulation to fill in memory deficits.

345.   The answer is A. *(Kaplan, ed 5. pp 203–204, 694–695.)* Delirium tremen can occur when a person stops drinking after prolonged use of alcohol. It is a hypermetabolic state that is associated with tachycardia, fever, tremulousness, and increased blood pressure. Affected persons are confused, are disoriented to time and place, and often have visual, tactile, or olfactory hallucinations. Symptoms usually last from 3 to 7 days. The mortality is significant in untreated persons.

346.   The answer is D. *(Schuckit, ed 3. p 154.)* Marijuana has been clearly demonstrated to decrease judgment, impair ability to estimate time and distance, and impair motor function. As with alcohol, these effects make accidents one of the major dangers of smoking marijuana. These two substances may also potentiate each other. Up to 17 percent of drivers in fatal accidents have tested positive for cannabinols. Driving ability is significantly affected for up to 8 h after smoking, and the ability of experienced pilots to fly is significantly decreased for 24 h.

347. The answer is A. *(Schuckit, ed 3. pp 178-179.)* PCP may cause a life-threateni[ ] toxic reaction with a combination of both sympathetic and cholinergic overactivity. There are no specific antagonists to PCP, and treatment is predominantly supportive. Phentolamine is used to treat serious hypertension, and gastric lavage must be considered when the drug has been taken orally. Behavioral control is often best handled by chemical rather than physical restraint, and both haloperidol and benzodiazepines have been employed to accomplish this. Acidification of the urine to a pH less than 5.0 will decrease the half-life of PCP from 72 to 24 h. Acidification may be required for up to 2 weeks in the longer lasting toxic conditions.

348. The answer is C. *(Schuckit, ed 3. pp 208-215.)* Caffeine belongs to the xanthine group of drugs. It is capable of producing panic, anxiety, and a worsening of panic disorder and agoraphobia. The half-life of caffeine is short, and flashbacks are not encountered with this drug. Tolerance and dependence occur with chronic use, and sudden withdrawal is associated with rapid onset of headache, muscle tension, irritability, anxiety, and fatigue. Overdose can occur through excessive coffee drinking or prescription drugs containing caffeine. Symptoms of overdose include hyperstimulation, tinnitus, derealization, and even confusion and hallucinations.

349. The answer is E (all). *(Talbott, pp 339-343.)* Cocaine, LSD, amphetamines, and mescaline can all present with clinical symptoms suggestive of schizophrenia. Perceptual disturbances—including hallucinations, delusions (particularly paranoid), and illusions—are commonly seen in drug abusers. An important factor in helping to make the differential diagnosis is that substance abusers usually experience visual hallucinations, while schizophrenics complain of auditory hallucinations.

350. The answer is E (all). *(Stoudemire, p 248.)* Intoxication with cocaine is usually characterized by subjective feelings of euphoria, elation, excitement, and restlessness. The patient often displays pressured speech, and on examination there are signs of sympathetic stimulation. These signs include tachycardia, mydriasis, and sweating. With chronic use one may see suspiciousness or frank paranoid psychosis. When intoxication is at the overdose level, hyperpyrexia, hyperreflexia, and seizures result. Ultimately there may be progression to coma and respiratory arrest. Cardiac arrhythmias may be associated with sudden death.

351. The answer is E (all). *(Kaplan, ed 5. pp 686-687.)* Alcohol dependence is described by *DSM III-R* as the pathologic use of alcohol resulting in impaired social or occupational functioning. The need for daily drinking in order to function adequately and an inability to cut down or stop characterize pathologic use, along with blackouts and continued drinking despite serious physical disorders related to drinking. For the diagnosis to be made, either tolerance or withdrawal symptoms must be evident. Tolerance is the need for increased amounts of alcohol to achieve the desired effect or a markedly diminished effect with the same amount, and withdrawal is physical symptoms (such as morning shaking) with reduction or cessation of drinking.

352.   The answer is A (1, 2, 3). *(Stoudemire, p 248.)* Cocaine is a high-potency local anesthetic that appears to work by blocking nerve impulses through its effect on sodium conduction of nerve cell membranes. It is also a potent sympathomimetic, potentiating the actions of catecholamines in the autonomic nervous system. This results in the characteristic tachycardia, vasoconstriction, and hypertension. The agitation and arousal effects are largely due to the stimulation of the central nervous system via potentiation of the actions of such neurotransmitters as dopamine and norepinephrine.

353.   The answer is A (1, 2, 3). *(Stoudemire, pp 248–249.)* An "amphetamine psychosis," with symptoms strikingly similar to those seen in paranoid schizophrenia, can be seen in chronic abuse of cocaine or other sympathomimetic agents, such as amphetamines, methylphenidate, and other stimulants. The manifestations include agitation, paranoia, delusions, and hallucinations. Propranolol and haloperidol are among the drugs reported as useful in overdose.

354.   The answer is E (all). *(Kaplan, ed 5. pp 679–680.)* Glue is a favorite substance of abuse among children and teen-agers. Intoxication can produce aggressive behavior, hallucinations, and amnesia for the acute period. Other volatile substances, such as toluene, lacquers, and paint thinners, are particularly dangerous because of the risk of tissue damage from repeated use. Death from overdose can occur.

355.   The answer is B (1, 3). *(Stoudemire, p 249.)* Patients intoxicated with PCP often present because of violence and bizarre, excited behavior. On examination one frequently encounters eye signs such as horizontal and vertical nystagmus. Myoclonus and ataxia are also common. Physical examination usually demonstrates the presence of tachycardia and hypertension.

356.   The answer is C (2, 4). *(Kaplan, ed 5. pp 689–690.)* Alcoholism is clearly the most serious drug-abuse problem in the United States. In 1974, a federal report estimated the number of cases of alcoholism to be 9 million. The rate of consumption of alcohol in this country was nearly one-third higher in 1980 than it was in 1964. Although it is thought that higher alcohol consumption means a higher prevalence rate of alcoholism in a given country, a cause-and-effect relationship has yet to be shown.

357.   The answer is C (2, 4). *(Hales, pp 162, 171–172.)* The adverse changes associated with meperidine use are commonly dysphoria, irritability, and myoclonic twitches. As toxicity increases with the accumulation of the metabolite normeperidine, there may be seizures and delirium. This picture is often seen in medical and surgical patients being treated for pain. The condition is treated by changing to another narcotic, such as morphine, at an equianalgesic dosage.

358. The answer is A (1, 2, 3). *(Kaplan, ed 5. pp 659-661.)* Medication frequently is used to help narcotic-addicted people through the withdrawal process. The most widely used medication is methadone; in programs of methadone maintenance, the drug must be taken on a daily basis. Although their main usefulness is in the treatment of narcotic overdose through their ability to displace opiates from receptors, narcotic antagonists also have been used in the prevention and treatment of narcotic addiction. Unlike methadone, narcotic antagonists do not themselves exert narcotic effects and thus are not addictive. Clonidine suppresses some elements of opiate withdrawal.

359. The answer is D (4). *(Kaplan, ed 5. p 1434.)* Alcohol idiosyncratic intoxication (pathologic intoxication) is a condition in which a person, usually of a younger age, after drinking a very small amount of alcohol, behaves as though he or she had drunk a great deal more. The onset is typically sudden and dramatic, often with aggressive behavior toward self or others. The episode may last minutes to hours and is often followed by a period of sleep and then amnesia for the episode. This is an uncommon condition, and patients must be assisted in achieving abstinence to avoid further episodes.

360-363. The answers are: 360-E, 361-A, 362-C, 363-D. *(Stoudemire, pp 237-238.)* These terms are commonly confused or used ambiguously. Tolerance refers to a pharmacologic effect in which a larger dose of a drug becomes necessary over time to achieve the same effect. Dependence is a condition in which withdrawal symptoms occur if the drug is stopped, and these symptoms indicate loss of control and usually lead to further drug use despite adverse consequences. The term *addiction* is often confused with *dependence* and refers to a whole repertoire of behaviors that serve to maintain drug use. With respect to drugs of abuse, one may see both tolerance and dependence simultaneously. The addicted person is one who has a whole series of behaviors and other phenomena that span the spectrum of the biopsychosocial structure of human existence. For this reason, successful treatment programs must be very broad in their approach to the patient's biologic, psychological, and social problems.

Psychotherapies

DIRECTIONS: Each question below contains five suggested responses. Select the **one best** response to each question.

364. In psychoanalytic theory, the phenomenon of transference

(A) occurs only in the relationship between the therapist and the patient
(B) impedes the progress of therapy because it distorts reality
(C) makes it difficult to reconstruct the patient's past
(D) involves the unconscious imposition of the experience of a past relationship onto a present one
(E) is manifested primarily in the patient's dreams

365. True statements about hypnosis include all the following EXCEPT

(A) it is associated with an EEG pattern different from that seen in sleep
(B) in general it is a safe procedure
(C) hypnotizability increases with increasing degree of psychopathology
(D) there are tests that can indicate a person's ability to be hypnotized
(E) it is not generally appropriate for the treatment of psychotic disorders

366. The behavioral therapy technique of systematic desensitization typically involves all the following EXCEPT

(A) homework assignments
(B) interpretation of unconscious conflict
(C) relaxation training
(D) construction of hierarchies
(E) imagined scenes

367. The major therapeutic techniques employed in cognitive psychotherapy include all the following EXCEPT

(A) "collaborative empiricism"
(B) interpretation of unconscious motivation
(C) behavioral techniques
(D) identification of irrational beliefs and automatic thoughts
(E) identification of attitudes underlying negatively biased throughts

368. Of the following, the most
sophisticated test of neurologically
based cognitive impairment is the

(A) Rorschach
(B) Bender-Gestalt
(C) Minnesota Multiphasic Personality
Inventory
(D) Halstead-Reitan
(E) Hamilton Rating Scale

369. In the technique of behavioral
therapy known as flooding, patients
are exposed to what they fear

(A) in massive amounts
(B) in repeated small doses, rapidly
presented
(C) in symbolic form
(D) in a relentless interpretation of
their conflicts
(E) in one of the above methods

370. The development of a transference neurosis during psychoanalytic
treatment

(A) typically occurs in the final stage
of analytic treatment
(B) occurs only with severely neurotic
patients
(C) is therapeutically useful
(D) usually represents a repetition of
rebellious adolescent conflict with
authority
(E) involves negative but not positive
feelings toward the analyst

371. The psychotherapy of personality
disorders is made more difficult by the
fact that character traits are usually

(A) ego-dystonic
(B) ego-syntonic
(C) unrelated to conflict
(D) so difficult to identify
(E) unrecognized by important per-
sons in the patient's life

372. All the following are true statements about supportive psychotherapy
EXCEPT

(A) regressive transference is encouraged and interpreted
(B) it is generally used for healthy
persons in crisis or for patients
with ego deficits
(C) a major goal is to support reality
testing
(D) suggestion and reassurance are
employed
(E) there is an attempt to strengthen
defenses

373. In psychoanalytic psychotherapy
the occurrence of countertransference
is

(A) inevitable to the process
(B) almost always harmful to the
process
(C) a sign that the patient should be
referred to another therapist
(D) a sign that the therapist is excessively neurotic
(E) an indication that the therapist dis-
likes the patient

374. Client-centered psychotherapy stresses which of the following characteristics in the therapist?

(A) Unconditional positive regard for the patient
(B) Intellectual reasoning power
(C) Confrontational ability
(D) Sensitivity to unconscious conflict
(E) Ability to give reality-based advice

375. Psychotherapy of stress-response syndromes most commonly

(A) emphasizes early intervention
(B) involves long-term psychodynamic psychotherapy
(C) uses antidepressant medication to relieve despondency and grief responses to acute loss
(D) encourages patients to maintain their normal activities during the acute phase
(E) avoids attention to preexisting conflicts and developmental difficulties that rendered the person unusually vulnerable

376. Erik Erikson's concept of the life cycle is characterized by all the following EXCEPT

(A) eight states of ego development
(B) the epigenetic principle
(C) phase-specific developmental crisis
(D) personality development completed by the end of adolescence
(E) generativity

377. Cognitive psychotherapy tends to focus heavily on

(A) unconscious and repressed memories
(B) mistaken ideas and beliefs
(C) transference ideation
(D) projective identifications
(E) none of the above

378. The form of psychoanalytic intervention developed by Heinz Kohut stresses

(A) confrontation
(B) interpretation of resistance and defense
(C) developmental conflict
(D) developmental deficit
(E) cognitive development

379. A woman with anorgasmia is undergoing sex therapy as originally described by Masters and Johnson. All the following statements about her treatment are true EXCEPT

(A) the treatment would include readings and explanations regarding sexuality
(B) the woman might be encouraged to achieve orgasm by masturbating herself
(C) the husband would not be allowed to participate in the therapy sessions until late in the treatment
(D) the patient would be instructed not to have intercourse early on in treatment
(E) the approach is strongly behavioral in its orientation

380. In order to be treated successfully in psychoanalysis, a neurotic patient must have all the following attributes EXCEPT

(A) a reservoir of basic trust
(B) a capacity for reality testing
(C) a capacity for internalization
(D) an ability to tolerate a dependent position
(E) a minimum age of 20 years

381. Which of the following statements is true of the psychoanalytic psychotherapy of patients with severe oedipal conflicts?

(A) The therapist should be of the same sex as the patient
(B) The therapist should be a male if the patient is female
(C) The development of an intense transference should be avoided
(D) The therapist should de-emphasize sexual topics
(E) None of the above

382. All the following statements about interpersonal psychotherapy (IPT) for depression are true EXCEPT

(A) it is a brief, weekly psychotherapy
(B) it was developed for ambulatory, nonbipolar, nonpsychotic patients
(C) the focus is mainly on current problems, conflicts, wishes, and frustrations
(D) regressive transferences are encouraged and interpreted
(E) rational problem solving is stressed

383. Traditional psychoanalysis is commonly used in the treatment of persons affected by all the following conditions EXCEPT

(A) conversion disorders
(B) obsessive compulsive disorders
(C) personality disorders
(D) psychotic disorders
(E) certain perversions

384. All the following statements about interpersonal psychotherapy, as developed by Klerman and his colleagues, are true EXCEPT

(A) it is a short-term psychotherapy
(B) it is often combined with medication
(C) it was developed to treat patients with nonpsychotic major depression
(D) the primary emphasis is on conjoint treatment of couples and group psychotherapy
(E) it aims to improve interpersonal communication

385. If a person is late for therapy four times in a row, the therapist should

(A) make up the time at the end of the hour
(B) admonish the patient
(C) try to elicit the meaning of the behavior
(D) ignore the behavior
(E) refer the patient to another therapist

386. An appropriate therapeutic attitude toward the schizophrenic patient includes all the following EXCEPT

(A) respect for the patient's need for privacy
(B) a consistent approach to the patient
(C) a desire to rescue the patient
(D) a focus on the patient's assets as well as on the patient's pathology
(E) tolerance of negative or bizarre behaviors

387. In general, group therapy is intended to enable individuals to do all the following EXCEPT

(A) learn new models of behavior
(B) discover that their problems are not unique
(C) develop a sense of belonging
(D) develop "basic trust"
(E) change their behavior to comply with group models

388. Group therapy is LEAST effective for individuals who have

(A) major mood disorders
(B) anxiety disorders
(C) personality disorders
(D) neuroses
(E) schizophrenia

DIRECTIONS: Each question below contains four suggested responses of which one or more is correct. Select

A	if	**1, 2, and 3**	are correct
B	if	**1 and 3**	are correct
C	if	**2 and 4**	are correct
D	if	**4**	is correct
E	if	**1, 2, 3, and 4**	are correct

389. Correct statements regarding biofeedback include that it

(1) usually employs instrumentation
(2) is designed to facilitate self-regulation of bodily processes
(3) may be used to modify brain-wave frequencies
(4) is an effective treatment for fecal incontinence

390. True statements regarding hypnosis include that it is

(1) associated with sleep electrophysiology as determined by EEG criteria
(2) a form of intense, focused alertness
(3) a treatment method first employed by Freud
(4) possible with the majority of psychiatric outpatients

391. The cognitive model of depression holds that the majority of depressed patients

(1) take a chronically negative view of themselves
(2) interpret life experience in a predominantly negative way
(3) look to the future in a pessimistic way
(4) have symptoms and affects derived from negative cognitive schema

392. Treatments commonly used in agoraphobia include

(1) administration of tricyclic antidepressants
(2) psychotherapy
(3) behavior modification
(4) administration of monoamine oxidase (MAO) inhibitors

393. People who have homosexual feelings or fantasies

(1) are regarded as pathologic by mental health professionals
(2) have an axis I diagnosis of homosexuality in *DSM III-R*
(3) show much more psychopathology than persons with exclusively heterosexual fantasies
(4) may be married and exclusively heterosexual in their behavior

394. Placebos have been shown to

(1) be frequently effective in the treatment of endogenous depression
(2) be frequently effective in the treatment of neurotic symptoms
(3) be frequently effective in controlling the primary symptoms of schizophrenia
(4) have potentially significant side effects when used to treat persons with psychiatric disorders

395. Studies of individual outpatient psychotherapy of schizophrenia have shown that

(1) psychotherapy often assists social rehabilitation
(2) psychotherapy alone is significantly less effective than antipsychotic drug treatment alone
(3) psychotherapy alone usually has little effect on acute symptoms
(4) psychotherapy plus drug treatment is most effective in preventing relapse

396. Existential psychotherapy is associated with

(1) a search for the meaning of a person's life
(2) an emphasis on past development
(3) spiritual values
(4) a theory of psychopathology

397. Day hospital programs play an important therapeutic role as

(1) an alternative to inpatient care
(2) a transition from inpatient care
(3) an alternative to outpatient care
(4) an alternative to nursing home care for the elderly

398. According to psychoanalytic dream theory, dreams can be described by which of the following statements?

(1) They often express transference wishes
(2) They are disguised and condensed expressions of unconscious mental content
(3) They have meaning in relation to the life of the dreamer
(4) They frequently involve the events of the preceding day

399. Psychoanalytic psychotherapies are characterized by a strong emphasis on the importance of which of the following?

(1) Unconscious motivation of behavior
(2) Precise descriptive diagnosis
(3) Concern with psychological defenses
(4) Phenomenology of symptoms

400. Violent behavior can be described by which of the following statements?

(1) It usually is committed by persons who have been exposed to violence in the past
(2) It can be lessened by individual and family psychotherapy
(3) It frequently is associated with alcohol intoxication
(4) Its occurrence can be predicted accurately by careful assessment of violence-prone persons

SUMMARY OF DIRECTIONS

A	B	C	D	E
1, 2, 3 only	1, 3 only	2, 4 only	4 only	All are correct

401. Normal grief reactions are characterized by which of the following statements?

(1) They typically begin with a state of emotional numbness or blunting

(2) They are usually worse if preceded by a period of anticipatory grief

(3) They are associated with increased rates of illness and death among bereaved persons

(4) The use of antidepressant medication effectively shortens the symptomatic period

402. Although the treatment of schizophrenia remains a controversial matter, current research focusing on methods of therapy suggests that

(1) intensive insight-oriented psychotherapy is an effective treatment of acutely psychotic patients

(2) a maintenance neuroleptic drug regimen is effective in preventing recurrence of psychosis in many patients

(3) social and psychological treatments add little or nothing to effective pharmacologic treatments

(4) phenothiazines are significantly more effective than placebo

403. A token economy involves which of the following therapeutic principles?

(1) Systematic desensitization

(2) Extinction

(3) Reciprocal inhibition

(4) Operant conditioning

404. The use of marital therapies generally is contraindicated if

(1) one or both partners have secrets they do not want revealed

(2) one or both partners are extremely paranoid

(3) one partner is anxious or fearful and refuses to participate

(4) one partner has a history of psychosis

405. Therapeutic measures used during brief psychotherapy can include

(1) crisis intervention

(2) use of psychotropic medication

(3) anxiety-suppressing techniques

(4) anxiety-provoking techniques

406. Important components of the psychoanalytic interpretive process include

(1) transference

(2) dream interpretation

(3) an understanding of current patient conflicts

(4) timing of the analyst's interpretation

407. Resistance that develops during analysis can be described by which of the following statements?

(1) It may be manifested by acting out
(2) It encompasses all the defensive operations presented by the patient
(3) It may be ego-alien or ego-syntonic
(4) It is easily recognized

408. In most sex therapies, treatment of premature ejaculation involves which of the following techniques?

(1) Sensate focus
(2) Stop-start technique
(3) Squeeze technique
(4) Use of anesthetic ointments

409. Behavior therapy employs which of the following techniques?

(1) Flooding
(2) Systematic desensitization
(3) Modeling
(4) Relaxation training

410. In contrast to adults in therapy, children in therapy tend to

(1) be highly motivated about their therapy
(2) develop early global transference reactions
(3) prefer internal resolution of problems
(4) show limited capacity for self-observation

411. "Working through" is characterized by

(1) a repetitive process
(2) understanding of the historical development of a defense
(3) discovery of the purpose of a defense
(4) development of new defenses

DIRECTIONS: The group of questions below consists of lettered headings followed by a set of numbered items. For each numbered item select the one lettered heading with which its most closely associated. Each lettered heading may be used once, more than once, or not at all.

Questions 412–415

For each patient described, select the most appropriate therapeutic intervention.

(A) Psychoanalysis
(B) Brief individual psychotherapy
(C) Community meeting
(D) Behavior therapy
(E) Family therapy

412. A young woman with no previous psychiatric history develops an incapacitating fear of driving after being involved in a minor automobile accident

413. A 40-year-old married man, a successful businessman with a satisfying family life, is preoccupied with thoughts of becoming involved with a younger woman. He has no prior psychiatric history and no other complaints

414. A 16-year-old girl begins acting out sexually. Her school performance deteriorates. These symptoms coincide with the onset of frequent arguments between her parents, who have been threatening marital separation

415. An intelligent 25-year-old single woman, who has a successful career, complains of multiple failed relationships with men, unhappiness, and a wish "to sort out my life." A previous experience in individual psychotherapy had been somewhat helpful

Psychotherapies

Answers

364. The answer is D. *(Michels, vol 1, chap 8, pp 6-7.)* Transference is a ubiquitous phenomenon, but it is especially prominent in psychoanalytic therapies because they are conducted so as to maximize its occurrence. The discovery of transference by Sigmund Freud was one of his most important contributions. Transference involves the patient's seeing and experiencing the present through "past-colored glasses," thereby making it possible to reconstruct the past and understand the origin of the patient's conflicts. While it certainly may color the patient's dreams, its predominant manifestations are in the interactions with the therapist or analyst in the course of treatment.

365. The answer is C. *(Kaplan, ed 5. pp 1501-1516.)* The hypnotic state is not identical to sleep, and sleep EEG patterns are not seen. The neurophysiology of the trance state is not well understood. While there is considerable controversy about the clinical usefulness of hypnosis in psychotherapy, it is a safe procedure when used in a professional manner. There are numerous tests of hypnotizability, and the ability to be hypnotized is not related to the degree of psychopathology. It is generally not employed with psychotic patients.

366. The answer is B. *(Kaplan, ed 5. p 982.)* The behavioral technique of systematic desensitization is typically used to treat patients who have learned (conditioned) emotional reactions, for example fears and phobias. The patient is taught relaxation, and a hierarchy of increasingly fearful images or situations is constructed. Often using imagined scenes, the patient proceeds up the hierarchy from the least feared to the most feared, learning to substitute relaxation for the previously anxious response. Exploring the unconscious and interpreting unconscious conflict are not a part of this type of treatment.

367. The answer is B. *(Talbott, pp 872-875.)* Cognitive psychotherapy is a directive and time-limited psychotherapy that aims to identify and eliminate negatively biased thinking so that the patient becomes more logical and reality-based. It was originally developed as an intervention for nonpsychotic depressed patients. The therapist and patient, by "collaborative empiricism," identify the patient's irrational beliefs and illogical thinking pattern. They then devise methods by which the patient can test the validity of these beliefs and cognitions. The treatment is structured and behavioral, and it is not involved with dream interpretation or other vehicles for exploring the unconscious.

368. The answer is D. *(Michels, vol 1, chap 7, pp 6–7.)* There are a number of cognitive and motor performance tests that have been developed to evaluate or diagnose patients with neurologic disorders and cerebral impairment. The Bender-Gestalt test of spacial relationships and constructional ability was one of the original and most widely used instruments. However, it cannot evaluate sufficiently the wide range of cognitive functions that may become impaired in organic brain syndromes. The Halstead-Reitan and the Luria-Nebraska tests involve sophisticated test batteries that evaluate a number of cognitive and psychomotor skills and may help to localize neurologic impairment. The other listed tests may at times suggest the possibility of organicity, but that is not their major focus of inquiry.

369. The answer is A. *(Kaplan, ed 5. p 982.)* In flooding, patients are exposed to whatever produces their fear in as massive a quantity and for as long a duration as can be tolerated. Ultimately the fear response begins to dampen, until the patient can no longer feel it. The stimuli can be imaginary or an in vivo exposure can be produced. This is a form of desensitization.

370. The answer is C. *(Kaplan, ed 5. p 1447.)* The transference neurosis typically occurs during the middle stage of analytic treatment and is associated with the patient's experiencing a psychological regression to earlier developmental times of conflict. Because of the transference, patients experience what is in essence a "substitute neurosis" in which their earlier wishes and conflicts are experienced vis-à-vis the analyst. This is therapeutically useful because it helps to bring forth important memories, feelings, and reactions that can be interpreted and ultimately resolved in the context of the relationship with the analyst.

371. The answer is B. *(Michels, vol 1, chap 31, pp 5–6.)* In the personality disorders, character traits are typically ego-syntonic. This means they usually cause the patient little personal distress, making motivation for change less likely. This is in contrast to neurotic symptoms, which are experienced as unwanted "foreign bodies." The patient's character traits often cause great distress to those who must live with them. Character traits are formed in response to developmental relationships and conflict, as are neurotic symptoms. They become part of the patient's style of living and relating to others.

372. The answer is A. *(Talbott, pp 878–882.)* Supportive psychotherapy is generally employed for crisis intervention, and with patients whose ego-deficits or life circumstance make other forms of therapy inappropriate or impractical. The therapist attempts to maintain a reality-based, problem-solving, concerned relationship that will augment the patient's ego strengths and defenses. Commonly this will include giving advice, reassurance, and suggestion and assisting in reality testing. The treatment is not structured to maximize the likelihood of transference distortions as, for example, in psychoanalytic psychotherapy. Regression would not be encouraged, either in the transference or in general behavior.

373. The answer is A. *(Kaplan, ed 5. pp 1448-1449.)* Countertransference refers to unconscious needs, wishes, or conflicts in the analyst that are evoked by the patient. These reactions might result in either positive or negative feelings about or responses to the patient. Countertransference has a definite potential to be harmful to treatment by interfering with objective judgment and reason. However, it is inevitably present in psychoanalysis and probably all forms of treatment. Often it serves the very positive function of alerting the analyst to subtle or covert patient behaviors, or of helping to provide insight into the patient's behavior and feelings. The only instance in which referral to another analyst is indicated would be when the first analyst is unable to resolve a countertransference that is an impediment to treatment.

374. The answer is A. *(Kaplan, ed 5. pp 1482-1495.)* Client-centered therapy was developed by the psychologist Carl Rogers. It was initially known as "nondirective" psychotherapy. It is based on the belief that people have great capacity for self-understanding and constructive emotional growth, which can be realized in the context of a special kind of relationship. This relationship is characterized by nonjudgmental attitude, caring, empathy, and unconditional positive regard.

375. The answer is A. *(Bassuk, pp 261-270. Michels, vol 1, chap 41, p 15.)* It is generally agreed that early intervention will help prevent stress-response syndromes from becoming chronic and will shorten the required treatment time. Brief psychotherapies, often dynamic in nature, are most commonly employed. Antidepressants are generally not indicated in the treatment of acute grief reactions. One must caution patients about continuing activities that require attention and concentration (e.g., driving, operating potentially dangerous machinery) during the acute phase, since these mental functions are often impaired. Crisis intervention may include helping the patient with preexisting conflicts that are associated with vulnerability, since one goal of treatment is to help the patient to be less vulnerable in the future to similar stressors.

376. The answer is D. *(Colarusso, pp 27-33. Talbott, pp 145-146.)* Erikson postulates that the life cycle consists of eight stages of ego development, commencing with birth and ending with death. The stages are based on the principle of epigenesis. Like the human embryo, personality development follows a predetermined sequence of steps that is governed by inner laws of development. Each developmental stage is characterized by a specific conflict during which opposing psychosocial attitudes vie for ascendancy. This creates a specific developmental crisis, the resolution of which allows each person to move on to the next developmental stage. Unlike Freud, who was primarily concerned with childhood psychosexual development, Erikson believes that personality develops throughout life. Generativity refers to central tasks of Erikson's stage of adulthood. These include caring for, and training, the next generation, betterment of society, and the production of ideas through one's work.

377. The answer is B. *(Kaplan, ed 5. pp 1541–1550.)* Cognitive therapy is usually an active, structured, time-limited form of therapy. It is based on the premise that the way we process information and structure our experiences determines how we think and feel. The patient is helped to identify, test the reality of, and correct distorted and dysfunctional beliefs that distort cognitions. This leads to more realistic and adaptive information processing and, therefore, improvements in symptoms and behavior.

378. The answer is D. *(Kaplan, ed 5. pp 366–367.)* Heinz Kohut began his career a Freudian psychoanalyst, but later departed from classical theory to found what sometimes known as "self-psychology." He was less concerned with resistance, defense, and conflict than he was with developmental deficits that left lasting scars in the areas of self-cohesion and self-esteem. Important among these deficits were failures in such things as empathy and mirroring by which a child develops a sense of worth.

379. The answer is C. *(Talbott, pp 934–935.)* Masters and Johnson's therapy for anorgasmia is basically a behavioral approach to the treatment of sexual dysfunction, though some therapists include psychodynamic considerations. This is a couples-oriented approach, in which both partners participate from the beginning of treatment. In conjoint interviews they are encouraged to discover the nature of the problem, to understand each other's sexual experience, to dispel myths and inaccuracies about sex, and to become comfortable with sexual enjoyment. This may include encouraging solitary sexual pleasuring in which there is less anxiety provoked and then progressing to a graded series of exercises in which the couple becomes more comfortable with pleasuring each other. They are instructed not to have intercourse until late in the treatment, thereby removing a major source of anxiety regarding performance.

380. The answer is E. *(Kaplan, ed 5. pp 1454–1455.)* Criteria for the analyzability of a person's neurosis include all the following: the ability to test reality; a sense of trust in the therapist as well as in oneself to face unpleasant issues; the ability to tolerate dependence; the capacity to internalize experience; and the motivation to pursue an unknown course. Although the above qualities suggest the presence of a certain degree of maturity, analysis can be undertaken in adolescence.

381.   The answer is E. *(Michels, vol 1, chap 8, pp 1–13.)* There is nothing about ∞ 'ipal conflict that in and of itself would dictate the need for a therapist of the same or opposite sex. The patient will experience a transference independent of the sex of the analyst, for example, a mother-transference to a male analyst. Since psychoanalytic psychotherapy uses transference as a major vehicle to both uncover and then resolve conflict, one would certainly not discourage the development of transference. Similarly, it would not further the therapeutic work to de-emphasize sexual topics since they are important to oedipal conflict and therefore its resolution.

382.   The answer is D. *(Kaplan, ed 5. pp 1559–1560.)* Interpersonal psychotherapy (IPT) was developed for the brief (generally 12 to 16 weeks) treatment of ambulatory, nonpsychotic, depressed patients. It is based on the premise that interpersonal problems are commonly associated with acute depression. Examples would be abnormal grief reactions, role disputes, role transitions, and interpersonal deficits such as self-defeating patterns of relationships. The focus of the treatment is mostly on the here and now, with less attention paid to early developmental considerations. The therapeutic relationship is structured as an active collaboration.

383.   The answer is D. *(Kaplan, ed 5. pp 1454–1455.)* Psychoanalysis is a commonly used treatment for persons who have long-standing neurotic problems or character disorders. These problems include conversion disorders, phobias, obsessive compulsive neuroses, and certain perversions. Generally, persons who are psychotic or addicted to drugs or alcohol have underlying pathology too severe to withstand the demands of analysis. There are, of course, exceptions.

384.   The answer is D. *(Talbott, pp 868–869.)* Interpersonal psychotherapy is a brief treatment focusing on interpersonal problems and was developed for patients with nonpsychotic major depression. It is an individual psychotherapy aiming to improve communication and reality testing, clarify feeling states, and facilitate interpersonal skills. It is usually combined with antidepressant medication. While the treatment is based on psychodynamic theory, the focus is on current interpersonal events rather than intrapsychic issues.

385.   The answer is C. *(Talbott, pp 856–860.)* Lateness is a characteristic resistance and often has the goal of avoiding unpleasant or disturbing issues in therapy. If lateness occurs repeatedly during therapy, the therapist should explore the meaning of the behavior with the patient. Persistence on the part of the therapist, despite a myriad of excuses offered by a patient, often results in a precise determination of the reasons behind the lateness.

386.   The answer is C. *(Kaplan, ed 5. pp 806–810.)* Therapists' attitudes toward the schizophrenic patient are a central aspect of therapeutic technique. If therapists feel they must rescue the schizophrenic patient, negative therapeutic reactions may result. Therapists should be more concerned with being of use to those patients. Important aspects of therapists' attitudes include their consistency and availability; respect for the patient; valuing the patient's autonomy; an ability to focus on the patient's assets; tolerance for negative, bizarre, and incomprehensible behavior; and therapeutic optimism.

387. The answer is D. *(Kaplan, ed 5. pp 1520-1522.)* Many processes important to group therapy have been described. Cohesion is a fundamental process by which members develop a sense of belonging or loyalty. The group may draw on an individual's desire to "belong" when it exerts group pressure to initiate change in the individual. The group also provides a variety of models of behavior that group members may imitate. By universalization, a phenomenon common to groups, members learn that others have problems similar to their own. The goal is not to suppress individuality, but to help the patient understand how his or her individuality affects others, and vice versa. Primitive defects in "basic trust" are usually not appropriately treated by group psychotherapy.

388. The answer is A. *(Kaplan, ed 5. pp 1522-1525.)* Group therapy has been helpful in the treatment of patients who have a wide range of neurotic, psychotic, and personality disorders. Persons who have major mood disorders, however, are helped least by group therapy. Not only do severely depressed individuals, especially those who are suicidal, require more support and attention than is available in groups, but group therapy itself may aggravate symptoms of depression. Manic individuals tend to disrupt groups and usually are too restless to derive much benefit from group therapy. However, once their acute mania is controlled, they can profit from group treatment.

389. The answer is E (all). *(Michels, vol 2, chap 109, pp 4-11.)* Biofeedback usually employs instrumentation designed to provide the patient with visual or auditory feedback regarding physiologic processes. For example, the electroencephalograph may be designed so as to emit a designated tone when alpha waves are achieved through relaxation. The electromyograph might be used to monitor activity in a specific group of muscles, with a visual or auditory signal that is proportional to the degree of relaxation achieved by the patient. Biofeedback has proved to be a useful adjunctive treatment in such conditions as migraine, hypertension, and chronic pain. In the case of headache due to muscle contraction, and for fecal incontinence due to sphincter incompetence or impaired ability to perceive rectal distention, it is often a treatment of choice.

390. The answer is C (2, 4). *(Kaplan, ed 5. pp 1501-1505.)* Hypnosis is best described as a state of intense, focused alertness with a constriction of peripheral awareness. The EEG during a hypnotic trance shows that the brain is experiencing resting arousal. The use of hypnosis by healers dates back centuries. Early in his studies of the unconscious, Freud employed hypnosis to help patients reexperience and abreact early life trauma. He soon abandoned it in favor of analysis of the transference. It is believed that about two-thirds of psychiatric outpatient populations are hypnotizable.

391. The answer is E (all). *(Kaplan, ed 5. pp 1541–1543.)* Cognitive theory relates the development of psychiatric symptoms and syndromes to habitual errors in thinking (cognition). The depressed person is viewed as one whose symptoms and affects are the logical outcome of negative cognitive patterns. Self, experience, and future are viewed through "negative colored glasses." Cognitions are developed early in life and may be activated by a life situation or stress.

392. The answer is E (all). *(Michels, vol 1, chap 33, pp 11– 13.)* The most common treatment for agoraphobia combines drugs with behavior modification or psychotherapy or both. Drugs that have proved particularly useful are the tricyclic antidepressants, the monoamine oxidase (MAO) inhibitors, and alprazolam. Antidepressant medication helps to block the occurrence of spontaneous panic attacks, and alprazolam may also have an effect on anticipatory anxiety. Psychotherapy, often supportive in nature, and behavioral techniques are used to help the patient reenter phobic situations and decondition their anticipatory anxiety and avoidance.

393. The answer is D (4). *(Michels, vol 1, chap 45, pp 4–7.)* DSM III-R reflects the current view of most mental health professionals that homosexuality per se should not be regarded as a form of psychopathology. It is not listed as a mental disorder on axis I or II. The term *ego-dystonic homosexuality* is sometimes used t describe those who have unwanted homosexual arousal and who wish to increase heterosexual arousal. There are more similarities than differences between homosexuals and heterosexuals with regard to most categories of psychopathology. There are many people who feel an inner identity as a homosexual, but live an exclusively heterosexual life with regard to behavior. There are also many people whose inner identity is heterosexual, but who have homosexual fantasies that may or may not be reflective of sexual or nonsexual conflict.

394. The answer is C (2, 4). *(Kaplan, ed 5. p 1686. Michels, vol 3, chap 45, pp 8–9.)* Placebos are pharmacologically inert substances that the user believes are potent drugs. Placebos have been shown to be effective in relieving a variety of neurotic symptoms, including anxiety and depression. They often produce side effects, such as weakness, headache, and gastrointestinal symptoms. Placebo effects are influenced strongly by the attitudes and expectations of both physician and patient. Primary schizophrenic symptoms and endogenous depression do not respond to placebos.

395. The answer is C (2, 4). *(Kaplan, ed 5. pp 804–805)* Psychotherapy alone has been found to be less effective than drug treatment alone. Drug treatment in conjunction with psychotherapy appears to provide the best protection against recurrence of psychotic symptoms. Psychotherapy may have an adverse effect on some withdrawn schizophrenic patients and usually does little to resolve acute psychotic symptoms; however, it does assist social rehabilitation.

396.   The answer is B (1, 3). *(Kaplan, ed 5. p 2141.)* Existential psychotherapy departs from traditional psychiatry in that emphasis is placed on a person's own sense of the meaning of his or her life rather than on psychopathology and past development. Spiritual values also are important in existential psychotherapy. Exponents of this view suggest that each individual determines his or her own nature by a constant act of self-definition for which the individual is solely responsible.

397.   The answer is E (all). *(Kaplan, ed 5. pp 2086-2087.)* Psychiatric patients in any hospital programs spend their daytime hours in a hospital setting but go home during evenings and weekends. Day hospital programs may provide a useful transition from inpatient care for partially stabilized patients who are not yet fully ready to return to the community. For selected patients, a day hospital may be a more effective treatment setting than an inpatient facility. Similarly, a day hospital may be more effective than regular outpatient treatment for certain chronically psychotic patients and may be a valuable alternative to nursing home placement for many older persons.

398.   The answer is E (all). *(Kaplan, ed 5. pp 367-369.)* Psychoanalysis makes frequent use of dream analysis as a therapeutic tool to explore a person's unconscious thoughts. Psychoanalytic dream theory views dreams as distorted, disguised, and condensed expressions of the dreamer's unconscious wishes that permit unacceptable wishes to be fulfilled in the form of "hallucinations" during sleep. Thus, dreams contain valuable, though disguised, clues to the unconscious mental life of the dreamer. Recent experience often appears in dreams; this "day residue" is thought to be relatively neutral material used to construct the dream, the symbolic and thematic content of which is unconsciously motivated. Dreams often express the unfolding of the transference neurosis.

399.   The answer is B (1, 3). *(Kaplan, ed 5. pp 1916-1917.)* A variety of different psychotherapies are based on psychodynamic principles. These therapies include psychoanalysis, psychoanalytic psychotherapy, relationship therapy, some supportive therapies, and others. Psychodynamic principles focus on the forces and motivations underlying human thought, feeling, and action. In particular, they are concerned with unconscious motivation in psychopathologic experience and behavior. This concern is reflected in part in the attention dynamic therapists give to the resistances and psychological defenses of their patients. In contrast to dynamic psychiatry, descriptive psychiatry emphasizes precise diagnosis and careful observation of symptoms and behavior.

400. The answer is A (1, 2, 3). *(Michels, vol 2, chap 95, pp 7–8; vol 3, chap 32, pp 13–14.)* Violent behavior, especially when impulsive or irrational, frequently is associated with mental illness. Violent persons typically have been exposed to a culture that endorses violence or were raised in a family in which violence was common. Intoxicated persons frequently exaggerate the hostile intentions of others and misjudge the consequences of violent acts. Repeated studies have demonstrated a high correlation between alcohol intoxication and violence. Individual and family treatment can help to resolve the conflicts and alter the patterns of behavior that can lead to violent outbursts. Although previous episodes of violent behavior and other factors increase the likelihood of violence, the occurrence of violent behavior is very difficult to predict. Psychiatrists are often unable to predict accurately whether a person is likely to commit violent acts and have tended to overpredict violence markedly.

401. The answer is B (1, 3). *(Kaplan, ed 5. pp 1345–1348.)* Normal grief reactions typically begin with a period of shock and numbness, followed by a period of yearning and protest. The next, final phase is one of apathy and aimlessness. Anticipatory grief may reduce the severity of grief reactions in some instances. Bereaved persons have an increased incidence of both physical and emotional illness, as well as a higher mortality. They may benefit from the judicious use of sedatives and antianxiety agents, but pharmacologic suppression of the symptoms of mourning can be harmful.

402. The answer is C (2, 4). *(Kaplan, ed 5. pp 777–781, 1571.)* Recent research suggests that neuroleptic medications are effective in the treatment of acute psychosis and important in the prevention of relapse for a significant minority of schizophrenic patients. In double-blind studies, neuroleptics repeatedly have been shown to be more effective than placebo. Social and psychological interventions add significantly to the overall effectiveness of comprehensive treatment of schizophrenic patients. There is little evidence to support the notion that intensive insight-oriented therapy is effective in the treatment of acute psychotic symptoms.

403. The answer is C (2, 4). *(Kaplan, ed 5. pp 1463–1470.)* A token economy is an example of a treatment based on principles of operant conditioning. Positive reinforcement is used to reward desired behavior. Because inappropriate behavior is not rewarded, its frequency decreases; this process is known as extinction. Desensitization and reciprocal inhibition are principles of classical conditioning, not operant conditioning.

404. The answer is A (1, 2, 3). *(Kaplan, ed 5. pp 1550–1553.)* Contraindications to marital therapy include the refusal of a partner to participate, the existence of secrets that cannot be revealed, the insistence of one or both partners on the need for a divorce, or a highly paranoid partner. A history of psychosis in one or both partners need not be a contraindication to marital therapy. Marital therapy may be the treatment of choice in selected cases of acute psychiatric disturbance precipitated by marital discord.

405. The answer is E (all). *(Kaplan, ed 5. pp 1564-1567.)* Brief psychotherapies can be divided into two basic treatment types: anxiety-suppressive (or supportive) treatments and anxiety-provoking treatments. Anxiety-suppressive techniques include reassurance, active intervention by the therapist, environmental manipulation, brief hospitalization, and the use of psychotropic medication. Anxiety-provoking techniques involve focused interpretive work with carefully selected, highly motivated patients. Patients in crisis may be treated with either technique, depending on the severity of their problems and their level of motivation.

406. The answer is E (all). *(Kaplan, ed 5. pp 1444-1452.)* In the interpretive process, the analyst gives meaning to those psychological events that are incomprehensible to the patient. Clarification of the patient's ambiguous statements is the key to interpretation. The interpretive process makes use of transference and dream interpretation and relates current patient conflicts to factors in the patient's past. Timing is critical; generally, an interpretation should be presented just before patients understand it on their own.

407. The answer is A (1, 2, 3). *(Kaplan, ed 5. p. 1448.)* Resistance refers to the behavior a patient presents when defending against impulses uncovered in therapy. All the defensive operations that a patient employs are included in resistance. Resistances may be either ego-syntonic or ego-alien, and some, including acting out, may be hard to recognize.

408. The answer is A (1, 2, 3). *(Kaplan, ed 5. pp 1054-1055, 1057.)* The success rate in the treatment of premature ejaculation tends to be quite high. The treatment involves both partners and begins with sensate focus, a series of exercises designed to increase awareness of pleasurable touch, sound, and sight. The "squeeze technique" is an exercise in which the penis is stimulated to the first sensations of impending orgasm and then strongly squeezed at the coronal ridge, causing partial loss of erection. The stop-start technique consists of stimulating the man to a point just short of inevitable orgasm; at that point, stimulation is halted until the sensation of impending orgasm disappears. The use of anesthetic ointments has proved unsatisfactory in the treatment of premature ejaculation.

409. The answer is E (all). *(Michels, vol 2, chap 77, pp 1-12.)* Behavior therapy is based on the work of Ivan Pavlov, Joseph Wolpe, and others. It focuses on observable patient behavior, rather than on inferred mental states. The principles of conditioning and learning are important theoretical foundations of this approach. Systematic desensitization, a key technique in behavior therapy, permits a patient to overcome anxiety by gradually confronting an anxiety-provoking stimulus in a relaxed state. Flooding is a technique in which a patient directly confronts an intensely anxiety-provoking situation, is "flooded" with anxiety, and remains in this situation until calm and able to experience a sense of mastery. Modeling involves the overcoming of anxiety by observing and imitating a model who is free of that symptom. Relaxation training is the most common tool used by behavior therapists as an adjunct to other techniques, such as desensitization.

410.   The answer is C (2, 4). *(Kaplan, ed 5. pp 1910-1913.)* In dealing with internal conflicts, children tend to choose alloplastic or externally manipulated adaptations rather than internal modifications. In addition, they have a limited capacity for self-observation. Although global transference reactions occur early in the course of therapy, the value of subsequent transference reactions is limited. Because children generally are taken to treatment by a parent or teacher, their motivation for treatment usually is less than that exhibited by adults.

411.   The answer is E (all). *(Kaplan, ed 5. pp 1450, 1454.)* The process of working through begins with the recognition by analyst and patient of the patient's defensive maneuvers. The analyst then demonstrates that the defense is historically determined and is used to evade some drive and prevent this drive from becoming conscious. The process of working through must be repeated many times because the patient soon presents new variations of the defensive behavior. This process seems to speed up, however, as more of these interpretative confrontations occur.

412.   The answer is D. *(Kaplan, ed 5. pp 263, 982.)* Systematic desensitization, which is a form of behavior therapy, is the most appropriate treatment for this woman. Systematic desensitization is used to treat classic phobias, but this technique as well as other forms of behavior therapy may also be of benefit in the treatment of other psychiatric disorders. It would be expected to be a good choice of treatment since the phobia appears to be unassociated with other complicating psychiatric problems.

413.   The answer is B. *(Kaplan, ed 5. pp 1564-1565.)* Patient selection is an important aspect of brief psychotherapy. Using psychoanalytic principles, the clinician attempts to select patients who are above average in intelligence, motivated, and able to think psychologically. Having a focused chief complaint, e.g., this man's interest in a younger woman, is also crucial. Given this man's good work history, family life, lack of previous psychotherapy, and focused complaint, brief psychotherapy is a suitable treatment. Were it to uncover other, significant problem areas, then a longer term therapy might be indicated.

414.   The answer is E. *(Kaplan, ed 5. pp 1537-1538.)* Family therapy is a treatment of choice because this girl's symptomatic behavior appears to be linked to her parents' marital difficulties. Individual treatment, which would address the girl's symptoms, would not alter the marital or family problems, nor would it allow the parents to explore the impact of their daughter's symptoms on the marital relationship.

415.   The answer is A. *(Kaplan, ed 5. pp 1454–1455.)* This woman is likely to be an appropriate candidate for psychoanalysis. She describes long-standing problems in heterosexual relationships. These are likely to be due to unconscious conflicts. In addition, she is unhappy with her life. Because previous psychotherapy helped but did not stop her symptoms, assessment for psychoanalysis is a reasonable therapeutic intervention.

Psychopharmacology and Other Therapies

DIRECTIONS: Each question below contains five suggested responses. Select the one best response to each question.

416. Which of the following statements regarding benzodiazepine receptors is true?

(A) To date, there has been only one type of benzodiazepine receptor identified
(B) Benzodiazepine receptors are all presynaptic
(C) Benzodiazepine receptors are measured using oxazepam
(D) Benzodiazepine receptors are all affected by gamma-aminobutyric acid (GABA)
(E) Benzodiazepine receptors have little stereospecificity

417. Which of the following drugs has shown the greatest efficacy in the treatment of obsessive compulsive disorder?

(A) Alprazolam (Xanax)
(B) Clomipramine (Anafranil)
(C) Propranolol (Inderal)
(D) Phenobarbital
(E) Lithium

418. All the following drugs are commonly used to treat anxiety disorders EXCEPT

(A) phenobarbital
(B) alprazolam (Xanax)
(C) buspirone (BuSpar)
(D) imipramine (Tofranil)
(E) phenelzine (Nardil)

419. All the following are capable of increasing plasma levels of lithium EXCEPT

(A) thiazide diuretics
(B) indomethacin
(C) fasting and low-salt diets
(D) phenylbutazone
(E) high intake of coffee

420. All the following statements about carbamazepine are true EXCEPT

(A) it is used in the treatment of mania
(B) it is used in the treatment of severe anxiety disorders
(C) it may cause fatal aplastic anemia
(D) it is potentially hepatotoxic
(E) it has mild anticholinergic activity

421. Which of the following drugs is a tricyclic antidepressant?

(A) Fluoxetine (Prozac)
(B) Nortriptyline (Pamelor, Aventyl)
(C) Phenelzine (Nardil)
(D) Tranylcypromine (Parnate)
(E) Clonazepam (Klonopin)

422. A 25-year-old woman gives a history of having used 30 mg/day of diazepam (Valium) for the past 20 months. Which of the following statements is most likely to be true?

(A) There is a small chance she is physically dependent
(B) She is almost certainly physically dependent
(C) She is probably not psychologically dependent
(D) She is probably not physically dependent, but is psychologically habituated
(E) Concern about physical dependency is not necessary at this dosage level

423. All the following statements about electroconvulsive therapy (ECT) are true EXCEPT

(A) the principal indication is for the treatment of severe depression
(B) it may be particularly effective in patients with delusional depression
(C) it may be of benefit in the treatment of manic excitement
(D) it is a procedure with a relatively high mortality
(E) it may be associated with impairment of memory

Questions 424–426

A 29-year-old woman is brought into the hospital by her husband after having charged her credit card to the limit while buying 40 pairs of identical shoes. Her husband reports she has not slept in 2 days and paces the house all night. Her speech is pressured and its content difficult to follow. Two weeks earlier she had been extremely depressed. The diagnosis of bipolar disorder, manic, is made.

424. Before starting the patient on lithium, all the following tests should be done EXCEPT

(A) BUN and creatinine
(B) chest x-ray
(C) thyroid panel
(D) ECG
(E) pregnancy test

425. The initial daily dosage of lithium is most often tested at

(A) 75 mg
(B) 100 mg
(C) 600 mg
(D) 1200 mg
(E) 1800 mg

426. For long-term control, therapeutic lithium levels are

(A) 0.4 to 0.8 mg%
(B) 0.8 to 1.5 mg%
(C) 0.2 to 0.4 meq/L
(D) 0.6 to 1.2 meq/L
(E) 1 to 1.5 meq/g

427. All the following symptoms are commonly associated with a drug withdrawal syndrome involving central nervous system depressants EXCEPT

(A) lowered pulse, respiration, and body temperature
(B) tremor
(C) grand mal convulsions
(D) muscle aches
(E) gastrointestinal upset

428. All the following are true statements about fluoxetine (Prozac) EXCEPT

(A) the usual starting dosage is 20 mg/day
(B) its action is believed to be particularly on serotonergic neurons
(C) sedation is the most commonly encountered side effect
(D) it is commonly used to treat depression
(E) there has been speculation that it may show promise as an anti-obsessional drug

429. The half-life of a drug refers to

(A) how long the drug will last unused
(B) how long it takes to produce the drug
(C) how long the drug will remain at least one-half active
(D) how long it will take to metabolize one-half the drug
(E) the temperature a drug must be kept at to keep it from losing half its potency

430. A double-blind crossover drug study means

(A) the subject does not know whether he or she is getting drug or placebo during the study and is not told after completion of the study
(B) the researcher does not know if the subject is getting drug or placebo and is not told after completion of the study
(C) the subject is not told what he or she is taking and is switched from drug to placebo in mid-study
(D) neither the patient nor the researcher knows whether drug or placebo is being used, and a switch is made in mid-study
(E) none of the above

431. Clozapine (Clozaril) is one of the newer drugs used to treat chronic and refractory

(A) obsessive compulsive disorder
(B) dissociative disorder
(C) panic disorder
(D) Alzheimer's disease
(E) schizophrenia

432. All the following are symptoms commonly associated with tardive dyskinesia EXCEPT

(A) lip smacking or lip sucking
(B) tongue movements
(C) facial grimacing
(D) fine tremors of the upper extremities
(E) choreoathetoid movements of fingers and hands

433. Which of the following antipsychotics is the most potent?

(A) Chlorpromazine (Thorazine)
(B) Thiothixene (Navane)
(C) Trifluoperazine (Stelazine)
(D) Haloperidol (Haldol)
(E) Thioridazine (Mellaril)

434. The tricyclic antidepressants are
effective because of their ability to

(A) block postsynaptic dopamine
    receptors
(B) inhibit dopamine release
(C) inhibit the reuptake of dopamine
(D) inhibit the reuptake of serotonin
    and norepinephrine
(E) inhibit the release of monoamine
    oxidase

435. Side effects seen with tricyclic
antidepressants include all the following EXCEPT

(A) dry mouth
(B) urinary retention
(C) involuntary muscle movements
(D) orthostatic hypotension
(E) constipation

436. All the following symptoms are
associated with neuroleptic malignant
syndrome EXCEPT

(A) hypothermia
(B) rigidity
(C) confusion
(D) autonomic dysfunction
(E) rhabdomyolysis

437. Side effects commonly associated
with tricyclic antidepressants include
all the following EXCEPT

(A) blurred vision
(B) diarrhea
(C) dry mouth
(D) urinary retention
(E) tachycardia

438. Which of the following psychotropic medications can produce psychotic delusions, manic elation, or
disorientation in some patients?

(A) Diazepam
(B) Lithium
(C) Amitriptyline
(D) Chlorpromazine
(E) Phenytoin

439. A man who has agitated depression is started on the following medications (in daily doses): imipramine, 150
mg; perphenazine, 32 mg; and benztropine mesylate (Cogentin), 2 mg.
One week later, his wife reports that
he has been unusually forgetful during
the last 4 days and that last night he
awoke unusually confused about
where he was. On physical examination, the man appears slightly flushed,
his skin and palms are dry, and his
heart rate is fast. He is slow to
remember the date and has trouble
concentrating. He showed none of
these symptoms during his appointment last week. The diagnosis is

(A) extrapyramidal syndrome
(B) neuroleptic syndrome
(C) schizophreniform psychosis
(D) toxic brain syndrome
(E) cerebrovascular accident

440. Which of the following statements best describes the development of tolerance during chronic administration of benzodiazepines (e.g., diazepam)?

(A) No tolerance develops
(B) Tolerance develops to the sedating effect but not to the antianxiety effect
(C) Tolerance develops to the antianxiety effect but not to the sedating effect
(D) Tolerance develops to both the sedating and antianxiety effects
(E) Tolerance develops only in persons who have addictive personalities

441. The duration of action of a single dose of fluphenazine decanoate (Prolixin Decanoate) is

(A) 30 min
(B) 2 h
(C) 3 days
(D) 2 weeks
(E) 2 months

442. The minimum daily dosage of chlorpromazine (Thorazine) needed to produce a therapeutic effect in most psychotic persons is

(A) 10 mg
(B) 50 mg
(C) 300 mg
(D) 800 mg
(E) 1500 mg

443. The antimanic effect of lithium usually is observed within

(A) less than 24 h
(B) 1 to 4 days
(C) 4 to 10 days
(D) 10 to 16 days
(E) 16 to 24 days

444. The mechanism of action of antipsychotic drugs currently is believed to involve blockade at receptor sites for which of the following compounds?

(A) Histamine
(B) Dopamine
(C) Acetylcholine
(D) Epinephrine
(E) Gamma-aminobutyric acid

445. Which of the following drugs has the most pronounced anticholinergic effects?

(A) Amitriptyline
(B) Perphenazine
(C) Chlordiazepoxide
(D) Lithium
(E) Desipramine

446. Severe reactions and death have been reported in persons who had been taking an MAO inhibitor and then were given

(A) chlorpromazine
(B) diazepam
(C) lithium
(D) imipramine
(E) phenobarbital

447. Which of the following drugs is LEAST sedating?

(A) Chlorpromazine
(B) Imipramine
(C) Diazepam
(D) Lithium.
(E) Haloperidol

448. During a 2-month period, a 72-year-old woman who has senile dementia becomes increasingly withdrawn, shows little interest in food, has trouble sleeping, and appears to become more severely demented. Her medical status is unchanged. Which of the following courses of treatment would be the most reasonable?

(A) Bedtime sedation to improve sleep
(B) Diazepam, 5 mg three times daily
(C) A trial of tricyclic antidepressants
(D) A trial of perphenazine, 4 mg three times daily
(E) None of the above, because her condition is untreatable

449. In the order presented, the medications thioridazine (Mellaril), chlorpromazine, perphenazine (Trilafon), and haloperidol (Haldol) are characterized by

(A) increasing hypotensive effects but decreasing sedative effects
(B) increasing hypotensive effects but decreasing extrapyramidal effects
(C) increasing extrapyramidal effects but decreasing anticholinergic effects
(D) increasing anticholinergic effects but decreasing hypotensive effects
(E) increasing sedative effects but decreasing anticholinergic effects

450. The first few weeks of methylphenidate treatment for children who have attention-deficit disorder may be marked by improvements in all the following areas EXCEPT

(A) attention span
(B) scores on achievement tests
(C) tolerance to frustration
(D) responsiveness to family and friends
(E) performance in school

451. In the treatment of persons in alcoholic withdrawal, chlordiazepoxide (Librium) commonly is used in daily dosages as high as

(A) 20 mg
(B) 50 mg
(C) 400 mg
(D) 1000 mg
(E) 2000 mg

452. The serum level of lithium at which therapeutic benefit levels off and side effects increase usually is considered to be

(A) 0.5 meq/L
(B) 1.0 meq/L
(C) 1.5 meq/L
(D) 2.0 meq/L
(E) 3.0 meq/L

453. Clinical response to an adequate dosage of tricyclic antidepressants typically occurs how long after initiation of treatment?

(A) 1 to 2 h
(B) 4 to 8 h
(C) 12 to 24 h
(D) 3 to 10 days
(E) 21 to 30 days

454. Physicians caring for persons who have taken an overdose of tricyclic antidepressants should pay special attention to which of the following clinical indicators?

(A) Renal output
(B) Cardiac rhythm
(C) Serum levels of bilirubin
(D) Bowel sounds
(E) Serum levels of glutamic oxalo-acetic transaminase (SGOT)

455. The various antipsychotic drugs currently in use are all about equal in terms of

(A) cost
(B) side effects
(C) milligram potency
(D) antipsychotic effectiveness
(E) antiemetic effectiveness

456. The daily dosage range of imipramine that is effective for the treatment of most depressed adults is

(A) 2 to 25 mg
(B) 10 to 100 mg
(C) 25 to 150 mg
(D) 75 to 250 mg
(E) 200 to 800 mg

457. Tricyclic antidepressants block the action of which of the following drugs?

(A) Chlorpromazine
(B) Guanethidine (Ismelin)
(C) Diazepam (Valium)
(D) Phenytoin (Dilantin)
(E) Quinidine

458. Gilles de la Tourette's syndrome is a childhood disorder that often begins with facial tics and progresses to multiple tics, grimacing, and spasmodic utterances. Patients with this disease are usually treated with

(A) chlordiazepoxide
(B) haloperidol
(C) methylphenidate (Ritalin)
(D) tranylcypromine (Parnate)
(E) protriptyline (Vivactil)

459. In elderly persons, increased confusion and paradoxical agitation are most likely to be associated with administration of which of the following sleep-inducing medications?

(A) Secobarbital (Seconal)
(B) Flurazepam (Dalmane)
(C) Chloral hydrate
(D) Chlorpromazine
(E) Amitriptyline

460. Epinephrine is contraindicated for the treatment of hypotension in persons taking

(A) diazepam
(B) lithium
(C) amitriptyline
(D) imipramine
(E) chlorpromazine

DIRECTIONS: Each question below contains four suggested responses of which
one or more is correct. Select

A	if	**1, 2, and 3**	are correct
B	if	**1 and 3**	are correct
C	if	**2 and 4**	are correct
D	if	**4**	is correct
E	if	**1, 2, 3, and 4**	are correct

461. Seasonal depression is often
treated by

(1) antidepressant medication
(2) neuroleptic medication
(3) light (phototherapy)
(4) carbamazepine

462. A woman is being treated with
medication for her schizophrenia.
Which of the following medications
would commonly be used to control
her psychotic symptoms?

(1) Haloperidol (Haldol)
(2) Chlorpromazine (Thorazine)
(3) Thiothixene (Navane)
(4) Lithium

Questions 463–465

An acutely psychotic woman is
being treated with chlorpromazine,
400 mg daily. After 7 days, the
woman's psychotic symptoms have not
abated.

463. During the first few weeks of
treatment the woman may develop
extrapyramidal symptoms. These may
take the form of

(1) an acute dystonic reaction
(2) akathisia
(3) a parkinsonian syndrome
(4) tardive dyskinesia

464. The woman begins to complain
of dry mouth, blurred vision, and constipation. As a result, her physician
should

(1) consider that her psychosis may
be getting worse
(2) adjust the chlorpromazine dosage
(3) administer an anticholinergic drug
(4) ask her if she has difficulty initiating urination

465. A week after initiation of treatment, physical examination of the
woman reveals cogwheel rigidity and
resting tremor. Her physician also
might expect to find which of the
following?

(1) Intermittent euphoria
(2) Hypokinesia
(3) Corneal opacities
(4) Micrographia

466. Medications produced from opium include

(1) morphine
(2) chlorpromazine
(3) codeine
(4) diazepam

467. Benzodiazepines, such as diazepam, have some degree of cross-tolerance and cross-dependence with which of the following drugs?

(1) Alcohol
(2) Narcotic analgesics
(3) Barbiturates
(4) Phenothiazines

468. Side effects that are relatively common during the first few days of lithium therapy include

(1) nausea and diarrhea
(2) blurred vision
(3) hand tremor
(4) masked facies

469. Endocrine effects of the phenothiazines include

(1) increased secretion of growth hormone
(2) galactorrhea
(3) weight loss
(4) amenorrhea

470. Diazepam can be described by which of the following statements?

(1) Its administration is the preferred treatment of persons in status epilepticus
(2) It is a better muscle relaxant than is placebo
(3) It can eliminate stage-4 sleep
(4) It is not useful as a hypnotic agent

471. Measures aimed at minimizing the long-term risks of tardive dyskinesia associated with antipsychotic drug use include

(1) careful observation for early detection of signs of tardive dyskinesia
(2) restriction of the chronic administration of antipsychotic drugs to those persons with psychosis or chronic anxiety
(3) discontinuation of antipsychotic drugs when signs of tardive dyskinesia are detected
(4) prophylactic use of anticholinergic drugs in persons who have shown parkinsonian signs

472. Lithium is clearly effective in the treatment of which of the following disorders?

(1) Schizophrenic psychosis
(2) Major depression
(3) Anxiety
(4) Mania

473. Imipramine is generally regarded as effective in the treatment of patients who have

(1) mania
(2) tic disorder
(3) psychosis
(4) panic disorder

474. Early central nervous system signs of lithium toxicity include

(1) seizures
(2) ataxia
(3) hyperreflexia
(4) dysarthria

475. A person taking a phenothiazine medication is likely to develop tolerance to which of the following effects of the drug?

(1) Sedation
(2) Lightheadedness
(3) Extrapyramidal reactions
(4) Antipsychotic actions

476. Major determinants of serious adverse effects in depressed patients receiving tricyclic antidepressants include

(1) elevated plasma levels of the drugs
(2) concurrent treatment with antipsychotic drugs
(3) concurrent treatment with non-psychotropic drugs
(4) advanced age

Psychopharmacology and Other Therapies

Answers

416. The answer is D. *(Michels, vol 3, chap 50, p 9.)* Recent research has identified selective receptor-binding assays for benzodiazepines, having found H^3-diazepam binding sites in brain tissues. These binding sites exhibit stereospecificity and are divided into two types. Type I is anxiolytic and anticonvulsant without being sedating. These sites are found postsynaptically and are primarily in the cerebellum and cortex. Type II is presynaptic, is found mostly in the hippocampus, striatum, and brainstem, and causes sedation. Both types are affected by GABA.

417. The answer is B. *(Kaplan, ed 5. p 1587.)* Clomipramine is a tricyclic drug, and its chemical structure resembles that of imipramine. It appears to have an antiobsessional effect that is not as readily apparent with other antidepressant drugs. Clomipramine has been studied in both children and adults, and its efficacy is thought to be related to effects on the serotonin system.

418. The answer is A. *(Kaplan, ed 5. pp 1579-1591.)* Phenobarbital was historically used to treat anxiety, but is rarely used today. There are other more effective antianxiety agents, such as alprazolam. Also, the barbiturates have a considerable potential for addiction and problems of withdrawal. Antidepressants such as tricyclics and monoamine oxidase inhibitors are often used to treat panic disorder, a buspirone is a newer agent used to treat chronic anxiety states.

419. The answer is E. *(Schatzberg, pp 123-124.)* When a patient is stabilized on lithium, and a thiazide diuretic is added in ignorance, the lithium level can double or reach toxicity. Low-salt diets and fasting can also decrease excretion of lithium, thereby increasing plasma levels. Indomethacin and phenylbutazone (nonsteroidal anti-inflammatory agents) have been reported to significantly decrease excretion of lithium. Clinicians should be alert to the possibility of a high intake of coffee interfering with achieving therapeutic levels of lithium.

420. The answer is B. *(Talbott, pp 827-828.)* Carbamazepine has been found to be effective in the treatment of acute manic episodes, as well as in the prophylactic treatment of mania. It is not used in the treatment of anxiety disorders. One problem with the use of this drug relates to its potential for hepatotoxicity and hematologic toxicity, including aplastic anemia. Since the drug has mild anticholinergic activity, some patients may complain of blurred vision, constipation, and dry mouth. Other complaints include dizziness, ataxia, and drowsiness.

421. The answer is B. *(Kaplan, ed 5. pp 1584–1585.)* Tricyclic drugs in common use include imipramine, desipramine, and nortriptyline. They are usually employed in the treatment of panic disorder and depression. While similar in their anti-depressant and antianxiety effects, they are associated with different side-effect profiles. For example, desipramine has less anticholinergic effect than imipramine, and nortriptyline is less likely to cause orthostatic hypotension.

422. The answer is B. *(Schuckit, ed 3. pp 19–36.)* The benzodiazepines are best used for short-term treatment (2 to 4 weeks). They are not effective over a long period of time, and one can expect a rebound increase in symptoms if the drugs are stopped. Benzodiazepines, and especially, diazepam, are very common drugs of abuse. The development of physical dependence relates to the drug dose and the length of time it is taken. Physical withdrawal has been reported with diazepam in the clinical dose range of 10 to 20 mg/day when taken over a period of weeks to months. This woman is probably physically dependent, and a drug withdrawal syndrome must be considered. Psychological dependency accompanies physical dependency.

423. The answer is D. *(Talbott, pp 836–841.)* In general, ECT is a relatively safe procedure. The morbidity and mortality are not significantly greater than for general anesthesia. The mortality is approximately one per 10,000 patients. Its principal indication is in the treatment of severe depression, particularly delusional depression and depression unresponsive to antidepressant medication. It is also used in elderly patients who cannot tolerate the side effects of antipsychotic or anti-depressant agents. ECT has been found useful in the treatment of acute manic excitement that cannot be otherwise controlled. Impairment of memory is a common but variable complaint of patients receiving this treatment.

424–426. The answers are: 424-B, 425-C, 426-D. *(Kaplan, ed 5. pp 1655–1662.)* Lithium is the drug of choice for bipolar disorders. Its advantages over neuroleptics include a greater degree of specificity and ease in monitoring plasma levels, and it does not produce tardive dyskinesia. Therapeutic blood levels for long-term maintenance are from 0.6 to 1.2 meq/L, and it has a serum half-life of about 24 h. Being a salt, it "competes" in the body with sodium and has effects on the heart, kidney, and thyroid. It can also cause birth defects. Unless indicated for another reason, a chest x-ray is not mandatory as a preadministration screen. Initial dosage is variable, but a test dose of 600 mg is often chosen to establish the regimen. The average adult usually requires 900 to 1200 mg/day for long-term control, and about 1800 mg/day for the treatment of acute mania.

427. The answer is A. *(Schuckit, ed 3. p 36.)* The drug withdrawal syndrome related to central nervous system depressants has a mixture of both physical and psychological symptoms. Patients often complain of gastrointestinal upset, muscle aches, and sometimes headache and malaise. The most common autonomic nervous system reaction would be increased pulse and respiration rates, labile blood pressure, and fever. Barbiturate withdrawal is associated with the danger of grand mal convulsions.

428. The answer is C. *(Schuckit, ed 3. pp 999, 1587, 1631.)* Fluoxetine (Prozac) was one of the most commonly prescribed antidepressants in the United States in 1990. Because of its effects on the serotonergic system, some clinicians have reported that it may have an antiobsessional effect similar to that of clomipramine. The most common side effects of this drug relate to nervousness and difficulty sleeping. The usual starting dose is 20 mg/day, and this is a sufficient treatment level for many patients.

429. The answer is D. *(Michels, vol 3, chap 45, pp 2–10.)* The half-life of a drug refers to how long it will take the body to metabolize one-half of the drug. Knowing the half-life is important in determining how often a drug should be administered. It is also helpful to know where a drug is metabolized. For example, drugs excreted via the renal system will be affected by any form of altered renal function. Organ pathology can greatly alter the normal half-life of a medication.

430. The answer is D *(Michels, vol 3, chap 45, pp 8–9.)* Double-blind crossover studies are done to control for individual differences in drug response and the placebo effect. They are conducted with neither the subject (patient) nor the researcher (physician) knowing whether the substance being taken is placebo or drug. This is double-blind. Crossover refers to changing from drug to placebo, or vice versa, in mid-study, again without knowledge of the subject or researcher.

431. The answer is E. *(Kaplan, ed 5. p 786.)* Clozapine (Clozaril) is a relatively new drug used to treat chronic and refractory schizophrenia. A significant number of patients using this drug have developed a potentially fatal agranulocytosis. For this reason it is generally not employed until it is established that the patient is unresponsive to the normally prescribed neuroleptics. A special system has been established to monitor patients on this drug.

432. The answer is D. *(Kaplan, ed 5. p 783.)* Tardive dyskinesia consists of abnormal involuntary movements. It is seen in some patients who have received long-term antipsychotic medication. Chewing motions, lip smacking or sucking, and tongue movements are common. The patient may demonstrate facial grimacing, and choreoathetoid movements of the fingers and hands are also seen and on occasion can extend to the trunk and extremities.

433.   The answer is D. *(Michels, vol 1, chap 55, pp 11–18.)* The potency of an antipsychotic relates to its ability to block postsynaptic dopamine receptors. In general, the more potent the drug, the less sedating it is. Haldol is a high-potency neuroleptic, many times more potent than Thorazine, Mellaril, Navane, and Stelazine.

434.   The answer is D. *(Michels, vol 3, chap 50, pp 10–11.)* Tricyclic antidepressants inhibit the reuptake of serotonin and norepinephrine presynaptically. Recent research regarding tricyclics has discovered that up-and-down regulation of adrenergic receptor sensitivity is also important. The antipsychotic medications are a different class of substances. They are believed to exert their effects through blocking of postsynaptic dopamine receptors.

435.   The answer is C. *(Michels, vol 3, chap 50, pp 11–13.)* Tricyclics, with their anticholinergic properties, can cause dry mouth, constipation, urinary retention, and orthostatic hypotension (a fall in blood pressure when sitting up). These side effects are commonly dose-related and subside to some extent with time in most patients. Movement disorders are sometimes seen with use of antipsychotic drugs, but are not usually associated with tricyclics.

436.   The answer is A. *(Kaplan, ed 5. pp 783–784.)* The neuroleptic malignant syndrome is associated with administration of antipsychotic drugs. It characteristically is manifested by fever, not hypothermia. It is also associated with confusion, rigidity, and autonomic dysfunction. Normally the condition resolves with discontinuance of the antipsychotic drug, but the mortality may be as high as 20 percent.

437.   The answer is B. *(Kaplan, ed 5. pp 1644–1648.)* Tricyclic antidepressants have anticholinergic properties. As a result they typically cause blurred vision, dry mouth, dizziness, tachycardia, and palpitations. They generally cause constipation rather than diarrhea. More serious side effects include urinary retention and paralytic ileus.

438.   The answer is C. *(Kaplan, ed 5. p 1647.)* Many drugs can produce disorientation as part of a toxic brain syndrome. However, the tricyclic antidepressants, such as amitriptyline, can stimulate psychosis in a schizophrenic patient or mania in a manic-depressive patient.

439.   The answer is D. *(Michels, vol 2, chap 111, pp 2–5.)* Phenothiazines, tricyclic antidepressants, and antiparkinsonian agents (such as benztropine mesylate) all have anticholinergic properties. The action of these drugs becomes additive when they are administered in combination. It is not uncommon for persons receiving such a combination to show evidence of a mild organic brain syndrome, including difficulty in concentrating, impaired short-term memory, and disorientation, which often is more noticeable at night. Dry skin and palms are especially suggestive of atropinism.

440. The answer is D. *(Michels, vol 3, chap 17, pp 7-8, 10.)* The minor tranquilizers or antianxiety agents, such as diazepam, are similar to barbiturates and other central nervous system depressants in that tolerance develops to both their sedating and their antianxiety effects. As a result, effectiveness diminishes with chronic administration.

441. The answer is D. *(Michels, vol 1, chap 55, pp 7-12.)* Fluphenazine decanoate is the decanoic-acid ester of fluphenazine (Prolixin). Esterification of fluphenazine slows its release from the injection site. The usual duration of action of intramuscular fluphenazine decanoate averages 2 to 4 weeks with maintenance treatment. Dosage must be individualized.

442. The answer is C. *(Kaplan, ed 5. p 1630.)* A number of controlled studies have demonstrated that chlorpromazine (Thorazine), when given in daily dosages of 300 mg or greater, was a significantly more effective antipsychotic agent than was placebo. At dosages below 300 mg, this effect was not demonstrated clearly, although other effects of chlorpromazine are noted at lower dosages.

443. The answer is C. *(Michels, vol 1, chap 61, p 19.)* The antimanic effect of lithium on manic patients usually is observed in 4 to 10 days. If a patient is agitated, sleepless, or otherwise unmanageable during the initiation of lithium therapy, an antipsychotic agent (either haloperidol or a phenothiazine) may be used.

444. The answer is B. *(Kaplan, ed 5. pp 36-39.)* Antipsychotic drugs block dopamine receptor sites. Blockade of dopamine receptors in the limbic system i believed to be responsible for the antipsychotic effects. Blockade in the basal ganglia results in the "extrapyramidal" side effects of the drugs.

445. The answer is A. *(Kaplan, ed 5. pp 1622-1623, 1646.)* The anticholinergic or atropinic side effects of the tricyclic antidepressants can be pronounced. Dry mouth, for example, is routinely produced by therapeutic dosages of tricyclic antidepressant agents. Among the tricyclic antidepressants, amitriptyline is one of the most potent anticholinergic agents and desipramine the least. The anticholinergic effects of the phenothiazines are less strong. Lithium and the benzodiazepines are not atropinic.

446. The answer is D. *(Kaplan, ed 5. p 1652.)* Severe reactions, even death, have been reported in persons receiving an MAO inhibitor who were given a high dose of tricyclic antidepressant. This observation has led to the belief that the two drugs might be a lethal combination. A waiting period of a week or more is indicated when switching from an MAO inhibitor to a tricyclic antidepressant.

447.   The answer is D. *(Kaplan, ed 5. pp 1660–1661.)* The only one of the major drugs used in psychiatry that does not produce some sedation or euphoria in normal subjects is lithium. This observation appears to be related to the clinical finding that persons receiving lithium therapy, unlike those taking phenothiazines or tricyclic antidepressants, seldom complain of feeling drugged.

448.   The answer is C. *(Kaplan, ed 5. pp 620–623.)* Depression in elderly persons, especially those who already have some evidence of dementia, may suggest deterioration of the organic process. The differentiation of progressing dementia from depression may be impossible. If the onset of symptoms is reasonably abrupt (1 or 2 months) and the patient has other signs suggestive of depression (e.g., changes in sleeping and eating habits) accompanied by motor retardation or agitation, depression should be considered. It certainly is preferable to consider a trial of antidepressants, which might be beneficial, rather than to assume a person's dementia is gressive and untreatable. Potential worsening of this condition, due to the side ects of medication, is a problem.

449.   The answer is C. *(Kaplan, ed 5. pp 1605–1606.)* The antipsychotic drugs listed in the question are arranged in order of increasing extrapyramidal effects and decreasing anticholinergic, hypotensive, and sedative effects. Knowledge of the position of a drug along this side-effect gradient is useful in selecting the most suitable drug for a given individual. It should be remembered, too, that individuals experience a variety of side effects for which they exhibit variable tolerances.

450.   The answer is B. *(Kaplan, ed 5. pp 1835–1836.)* Methylphenidate and the amphetamines, when effective, can lengthen attention span, reduce hyperactivity, and increase frustration tolerance in children who have attention-deficit disorder. As a result, school performance improves, and the children become more sensitive to family and friends. Although school performance is improved by the increased attention span, affected children already may be considerably behind peers in academic achievement. Therefore, it is necessary to place these children in grades appropriate to their level of achievement, and if perceptual problems persist, these children should be enrolled in special education classes.

451.   The answer is C. *(Kaplan, ed 5. p 697.)* Chlordiazepoxide (Librium) frequently is used in the treatment of persons in alcoholic withdrawal. Dosage must be sufficient to relieve tremors and agitation. Dosage will vary, but commonly will be in the range of 200 to 400 mg/day.

452.   The answer is C. *(Kaplan, ed 5. p 1656.)* The therapeutic serum concentration of lithium for manic patients is 0.6 to 1.2 meq/L. In maintenance therapy, a level of 0.6 to 1.0 meq/L usually is sufficient. At lithium levels higher than 1.5 meq/L, the incidence of side effect rapidly increases.

453. The answer is D. *(Kaplan, ed 5. p 1627.)* Improvement in the condition of a depressed patient receiving a tricyclic antidepressant at an adequate dosage often appears in 3 to 10 days, is usually present by 2 weeks, but sometimes may not occur until the third week. For this reason, many clinicians feel that an adequate trial of a tricyclic antidepressant requires at least 3 weeks of treatment. Although patients who have a partial response may continue to improve, those who have not responded to treatment at the end of 3 weeks either require treatment at higher dosage or need different treatment.

454. The answer is B. *(Kaplan, ed 5. pp 1644-1646.)* Cardiac arrhythmia, which sometimes can be fatal, is the most common dangerous consequence of an overdose of tricyclic antidepressant. For this reason, electrocardiographic monitoring is advised for persons who have taken a significant overdose. Physostigmine can be used to reverse the anticholinergic effects of the drug.

455. The answer is D. *(Kaplan, ed 5. pp 1604-1606.)* The antipsychotic compounds currently in use are generally equal in their antipsychotic effects when used in the appropriate dosage. Dosage varies because the drugs vary in potency on a milligram-per-milligram basis. Therefore, the primary factor affecting the selection of an antipsychotic agent is its potential for causing side effects. Cost and antiemetic effects also vary among these drugs.

456. The answer is D. *(Kaplan, ed 5. p 1634.)* The effective dosage range of imipramine for most patients is 75 to 250 mg daily. In a few persons, dosages above or below this range may be required because of unusual pharmacokinetics. A common error is to continue treatment at inadequate dosage levels.

457. The answer is B. *(Kaplan, ed 5. pp 1663-1664.)* Guanethidine (Ismelin) produces its antihypertensive effect after its uptake by peripheral noradrenergic neurons. Because tricyclic antidepressants block this uptake mechanism, guanethidine cannot reach its site of action.

458. The answer is B. *(Kaplan, ed 5. pp 1876-1877.)* Haloperidol has been reported to reduce symptoms by 90 percent in most people who have Gilles de la Tourette's syndrome. The dosage prescribed by clinicians ranges considerably. Ritalin is sometimes used to treat tic disorders.

459. The answer is A. *(Talbott, pp 1135-1136.)* Although any sedating drug has the potential for adding to the confusion of an elderly person, the barbiturates are most frequently associated with paradoxical agitation or excitement. Chloral hydrate and flurazepam (Dalmane) are useful in treating insomnia in older persons.

In the treatment of insomnia in an elderly patient who has either psychosis or depression, an antipsychotic or antidepressant drug may be indicated.

460. The answer is E. *(Kaplan, ed 5. p 1620.)* Chlorpromazine, through its alpha-adrenergic blockade, blocks the alpha-stimulating effect of epinephrine, allowing the beta-stimulating effect to predominate. Thus, instead of having a pressor effect, epinephrine produces hypotension. Hypotension in a person receiving chlorpromazine should be treated with volume expansion and administration of norepinephrine, which has alpha-stimulating but not beta-stimulating effects.

461. The answer is B (1, 3). *(Talbott, p 433.)* The syndrome of seasonal affective disorder often presents with the regular occurrence of major depressive episodes in the late fall or winter, with remission in the spring. Sometimes hypomania will appear in the summer. Patients are often treated with antidepressant medication, but tend to be poor responders. Exposure to several hours of bright artificial light (phototherapy) brings rapid and marked improvement to the majority of patients suffering from this syndrome.

462. The answer is A (1, 2, 3). *(Kaplan, ed 5. pp 778-779.)* Schizophrenia is a chronic psychotic disorder. It is responsive to diverse pharmacologic treatments. The mainstay of treatment for schizophrenia is the group of medications called antipsychotics or neuroleptics. They include the phenothiazines (Thorazine, Mellaril, Stelazine, Prolixin), butyrophenones (Haldol), thioxanthenes (Navane), and others. Lithium is the treatment of choice in mania, but is not commonly used to treat schizophrenia.

463. The answer is A (1, 2, 3). *(Kaplan, ed 5. pp 1622-1624.)* Extrapyramidal reactions during the first weeks of chlorpromazine treatment generally are divided into three categories. Acute dystonic reactions, the first category, often occur within the first few days of treatment and respond dramatically to antiparkinsonian drugs. Akathisia (motor restlessness), the second type of extrapyramidal reaction, may be difficult to differentiate from a worsening of the underlying psychosis; however, unlike the latter, akathisia usually will respond to a reduction in the dosage of the antipsychotic agent. Parkinsonian syndrome is the third category of early extrapyramidal reactions. Tardive dyskinesia is a syndrome that results from chronic use of antipsychotic medication over a period of years.

464. The answer is C (2, 4). *(Kaplan, ed 5. p 1622.)* Dry mouth, blurred vision, and constipation are common dose-dependent anticholinergic side effects of chlorpromazine. Administration of an anticholinergic, antiparkinsonian drug will exacerbate these symptoms. The presence of difficulty in initiating urination, which is another anticholinergic side effect, should be ascertained because it can lead to urinary retention.

465. The answer is C (2, 4). *(Michels, vol 1, chap 55, p 26. Wilson, ed 12. pp 2065-2067.)* The woman described has a parkinsonian syndrome, symptoms of which include rigidity, tremor, hypokinesia, and micrographia. In addition, she is more likely to have a masked expression or a lack of affect than euphoria. Corneal opacities, which are late in onset and are relatively uncommon side effects of the use of phenothiazines, are unrelated to parkinsonian syndrome.

466. The answer is B (1, 3). *(Kaplan, ed 5. pp 645-649.)* Opium is produced from the seeds of poppy plants. The dried exudate of the unripe seeds is powdered to produce alkaloids. The ones used in clinical medicine include morphine, codeine, thebaine, papaverine, and noscapine. The morphine content of opium is 10 percent. These drugs are potent analgesics with strong addictive potentials. Chlorpromazine (Thorazine) and diazepam are synthetic compounds; chlorpromazine is an antipsychotic and diazepam a muscle relaxant, anticonvulsant, and anxiolytic.

467. The answer is B (1, 3). *(Michels, vol 2, chap 90, pp 10-11.)* Benzodiazepines demonstrate some cross-tolerance with other central nervous system depressants, including alcohol, barbiturates, and nonbarbiturate hypnotics, such as glutethimide (Doriden) and methyprylon (Noludar). This cross-tolerance not only enables chlordiazepoxide to be substituted for alcohol in the treatment of alcohol withdrawal but also explains the potential for benzodiazepine abuse by people who have previously abused other central nervous system depressants.

468. The answer is B (1, 3). *(Michels, vol 2, chap 59, pp 10-11.)* Side effects occurring during the initiation of lithium therapy include nausea, vomiting, and diarrhea. Appearance of these symptoms usually occurs at the peak plasma level. Hand tremor is one of the most common side effects during maintenance treatment and may improve with low-dose propranolol.

469. The answer is C (2, 4). *(Kaplan, ed 5. pp 1625-1626.)* The phenothiazines have a number of endocrine effects. Galactorrhea or amenorrhea can result from the drugs' effects on prolactin and gonadotropins. Phenothiazines also reduce secretion of growth hormone and adrenocorticotropin. Weight gain is a common side effect of the use of phenothiazines.

470. The answer is A (1, 2, 3). *(Kaplan, ed 5. pp 222, 1580-1581. Michels, vol 2, chap 105, pp 6, 15-16.)* Diazepam is a treatment of choice for persons in status epilepticus and is effective in a high percentage of cases. Because it can reduce or eliminate stage-4 sleep, it is sometimes used to treat persons suffering from night terrors. In addition to its sedating action, diazepam can be used as a hypnotic. Diazepam is sometimes also used as a muscle relaxant. Some muscle relaxation may result with use of any central nervous system depressant.

471.   The answer is B (1, 3). *(Kaplan, ed 5. pp 1623–1624.)* The long-term risk of tardive dyskinesia can be reduced by restricting the use of antipsychotic drugs to those patients who require chronic antipsychotic treatment—primarily, patients with recurrent psychosis. In syndromes such as chronic anxiety, other agents are employed. Patients receiving chronic antipsychotic drug therapy require careful observation because the tardive dyskinesia syndrome may more likely be reversible if it is detected early and the antipsychotic agent discontinued promptly. Antiparkinsonian drugs play no role in the treatment of tardive dyskinesia; in fact, their use may worsen the syndrome.

472.   The answer is D (4). *(Kaplan, ed 5. pp 1656–1658.)* Several double-blind studies have demonstrated the superiority of lithium over placebo in the treatment of mania. Although there have been interest in and suggestive evidence for the usefulness of lithium in the treatment of bipolar depression, its antidepressant effect in major depression has not been fully established. Lithium is not generally used in the treatment of patients who have a schizophrenic psychosis and is not used to treat anxiety.

473.   The answer is D (4). *(Kaplan, ed 5. pp 970–971.)* Imipramine reduces the frequency and severity of panic attacks in patients who have panic disorder. It is believed to sometimes exacerbate mania or psychosis and is not used to treat tic disorder.

474.   The answer is C (2, 4). *(Kaplan, ed 5. p 1660.)* Early signs of lithium toxicity include confusion, lethargy, coarse tremor, dysarthria, vomiting, diarrhea, and ataxia. If these signs appear, lithium should be discontinued immediately so that the plasma level can decrease. Continuation of lithium treatment can lead to hyperreflexia, muscle tremor and fasciculation, seizures, coma, and sometimes death.

475.   The answer is A (1, 2, 3). *(Kaplan, ed 5. pp 781–787.)* Most people develop tolerance to sedation and accommodate to the lightheadedness associated with the hypotensive side effects of phenothiazines. Tolerance to extrapyramidal side effects, which develops within 2 or 3 months, sometimes allows antiparkinsonian agents to be discontinued. Because patients do not develop a tolerance to the phenothiazines' antipsychotic action, these drugs can be used for years in maintenance therapy.

476.   The answer is C (2, 4). *(Kaplan, ed 5. pp 782, 1646.)* Major adverse reactions, which interrupt treatment, are more frequent in patients over 60 years of age and in patients concurrently receiving antipsychotic drugs with the tricyclic. The antipsychotic-tricyclic combination is especially associated with increased "anticholinergic" side effects, which may may be mediated by central rather than peripheral mechanisms. Plasma concentrations of these drugs are not routinely elevated in patients having serious side effects.

Law and Ethics in Psychiatry

DIRECTIONS: Each question below contains five suggested responses. Select the one best response to each question.

477. When a subpoena is delivered ordering release of psychiatric records, the psychiatrist

(A) must release the records immediately
(B) may update and modify the records before releasing them
(C) may demand a judicial hearing before releasing them
(D) may release them only with the patient's permission
(E) may refuse to release them because of doctor-patient privilege

478. All states now have laws requiring the physician to report cases of

(A) heroin abuse
(B) drug addicts admitted to hospitals
(C) psychosis with hallucinations ordering violence
(D) child abuse
(E) pedophilia

479. When a patient's illness has resulted in an inability to understand and therefore manage personal or financial affairs, a guardian may be designated after the patient is declared incompetent by

(A) a family member with power of attorney
(B) a judge following a hearing
(C) a psychiatrist, after a thorough examination of mental status
(D) a spouse
(E) a hospital administrator upon the advice of a psychiatrist

480. The standard for criminal responsibility in most U.S. federal courts is the

(A) product rule
(B) M'Naghten rule
(C) American Law Institute test
(D) irresistible impulse test
(E) Currens test

481. Privileged communication means

(A) that psychiatrists have the privilege of disclosing information about a patient to other psychiatrists or physicians
(B) that the information revealed by psychiatrists at a probate hearing is handled as privileged
(C) that psychiatrists are granted by the court the "privilege" to disclose information about a specific patient
(D) that patients have the statutory right to prevent psychiatrists from disclosing confidential information
(E) none of the above

482. In the nineteenth century, due-process procedures for civilly committed patients were expanded as the result of the work and writings of

(A) Dorothea Dix
(B) Elizabeth Packard
(C) Lyman Beecher
(D) William Lloyd Garrison
(E) Isaac Ray

483. The landmark decision in *Tarasoff v. Regents of California* held that a therapist has an obligation to

(A) protect the confidentiality of information obtained during therapy
(B) warn the university when students are involved in any illegal activities
(C) report to university authorities the presence of a student who is involved in illegal drug sales
(D) warn the potential victim of a potentially violent patient
(E) give informed consent to patients of the student health center who are given neuroleptic medications

Questions 484–485

A psychiatrist is called in to evaluate a wealthy 85-year-old man who is drawing up a new "last will" and is concerned that it might be challenged after his death on the basis of possible reduced mental capacity.

484. The psychiatric evaluation would be for the purpose of determining the patient's

(A) sanity versus insanity
(B) testamentary capacity
(C) ability to distinguish right from wrong
(D) judgmental capacity
(E) insight

485. The essential components of a valid will include all the following EXCEPT

(A) the absence of any axis I diagnosis
(B) knowledge of the nature and extent of one's assets
(C) knowledge of relatives and natural heirs
(D) knowledge that a will is being made
(E) freedom from undue influence

DIRECTIONS: Each question below contains four suggested responses of which **one or more** is correct. Select

A	if	1, 2, and 3	are correct
B	if	1 and 3	are correct
C	if	2 and 4	are correct
D	if	4	is correct
E	if	1, 2, 3, and 4	are correct

486. The physician is not legally or ethically bound to continue treatment if

(1) dismissed by a patient who is believed competent
(2) the patient is given ample medication to last until he or she finds a new therapist
(3) there is suitable notice and assistance given to find a substitute therapist
(4) the patient is uncooperative with the treatment

487. The ethical issue underlying the principle of informed consent centers on whether or not the patient has *knowingly* consented. Essential elements of informed consent include

(1) the patient's competency
(2) the patient's ability to rationally understand
(3) the patient's knowledge of the circumstances of the treatment or research
(4) voluntary agreement without coercion

488. The principles of informed consent and the usual common-law elements of disclosure include

(1) the nature of the procedure or treatment
(2) the risks that are material, substantial, probable, or significant
(3) the anticipated benefits including probability of success
(4) the alternatives

489. Informed consent need NOT be obtained from

(1) patients involved in emergencies that threaten life or serious bodily harm
(2) patients legally committed to a mental hospital
(3) patients who waive decision-making and information disclosure
(4) patients who are clearly and manifestly psychotic

490. Tarasoff II, the second decision by the California Supreme Court, revised the original ruling by

(1) requiring the warning of only "identifiable" victims
(2) declaring immunity for the police
(3) requiring hospitalization of patients deemed dangerous
(4) finding a duty to protect victims, not just warn them

491. In 1843 Daniel M'Naghten was
tried and found not guilty by reason of
insanity. This insanity verdict resulted
in the

(1) establishment of the "good versus
evil" standard
(2) development of standards used by
many states
(3) establishment of delusions as the
sine qua non of legal insanity
(4) lifelong confinement of
M'Naghten in an asylum

492. Physicians have the duty to disclose risks of treatment to their
patients EXCEPT in instances where

(1) minimal risks are involved
(2) a medical emergency is involved
(3) disclosure would definitively result
in the deterioration of a patient's
physical or mental condition
(4) disclosure might cause the patient
to refuse treatment

493. Competence to stand trial is described by which of the following
statements?

(1) The U.S. Supreme Court has not
yet defined a standard
(2) It is possible for a defendant to be
competent for one charge and not
for another
(3) Mental status must be assessed
both at the time of the crime and
at the time of trial
(4) A person with a total organic
amnesia for the events of a crime
still may be judged competent

494. Psychiatrists who have sexual
relationships with their patients are

(1) in violation of the American Psychiatric Association's guidelines
for ethical conduct
(2) liable to malpractice suits, even if
the patient consented
(3) in jeopardy of having their license
revoked by their state medical
licensing board
(4) liable to prosecution for rape

495. Psychiatrists giving testimony in
court should know that

(1) their testimony must conform to
the "reasonable medical certainty"
standard
(2) they may give opinion testimony if
accepted as an expert witness
(3) they may give opinion as to the
ultimate issue to be decided by the
trier of fact
(4) they may not use lie detectors or
other such tests, which are inadmissible, to support an opinion

DIRECTIONS: The group of questions below consists of lettered headings followed by a set of numbered items. For each numbered item select the one lettered heading with which it is most closely associated. Each lettered heading may be used once, more than once, or not at all.

Questions 496–500

Match the following.

(A) M'Naghten rule
(B) Irresistible impulse rule
(C) American Law Institute: Model Penal Code
(D) Durham rule
(E) *Mens rea* elements

496. Psychiatric testimony should only be addressed to the issue of state of mind and criminal intent at the time of the crime

497. An insanity defense related to inability to know the nature and quality of the act being done, or that what was being done was wrong

498. An accused is not criminally responsible if the unlawful act was the product of mental disease or mental defect

499. A test of criminal responsibility that specifically excludes those conditions that may have associated sociopathic behaviors, such as some personality disorders

500. "A person is not responsible for criminal conduct if at the time of such conduct as a result of mental disease or defect he lacks substantial capacity either to appreciate the criminality (wrongfulness) of his conduct or to conform his conduct to the requirements of the law"

Law and Ethics in Psychiatry

Answers

477. The answer is C. *(Michels, vol 3, chap 31, pp 9–10.)* A subpoena does not require that the psychiatrist immediately surrender the psychiatric records. It cannot be enforced until there is an opportunity to appear before a judge in a hearing. This offers an opportunity to present arguments such as belief that the release of the information will be destructive to the patient or the family. By contrast, a court-approved search warrant by law enforcement officers does not provide such an opportunity for challenge.

478. The answer is D. *(Michels, vol 3, chap 31, pp 13–16.)* Respect for the patient's confidentiality is considered by all psychiatrists to be essential for effective clinical practice. Psychiatrists have traditionally resisted attempts to place them in the role of an informer. The American Medical Association and the American Psychiatric Association have endorsed an additional ethical obligation to society under certain circumstances. All states now have laws for reporting child abuse. Some states, but not all, require that users of certain drugs be reported as well as persons believed likely to commit violence. There are also jurisdictions that protect the confidentiality of addicts and drug-dependent persons voluntarily seeking treatment. There is no obligation to report the existence of a sexual disorder that might result in unlawful acts.

479. The answer is B. *(Michels, vol 3, chap 36, p 12.)* Guardianship can only be established by a judicial proceeding, and careful attention is given to assuring the patient's rights. The psychiatrist may be called upon to give testimony regarding competency, but only the court can appoint someone to make decisions on the patient's behalf.

480. The answer is C. *(Halleck, pp 214–224. Kaplan, ed 5. pp 2121–2122.)* Most U.S. federal courts presently use the American Law Institute (ALI) test, or a minor variation, to determine criminal responsibility. The ALI standard states, "It shall be a defense that the defendant at the time of the proscribed conduct, as a result of mental disease or defect, lacked substantial capacity either to appreciate the wrongfulness of his conduct or to conform his conduct to the requirements of the law." Many jurisdictions have appended a section that states, "The terms mental disease or defect do not include an abnormality manifested only by repeated criminal or otherwise antisocial conduct." This provision is designed to prevent persons with antisocial personality from offering an insanity defense. Recent decisions in some jurisdictions suggest that the federal judiciary may be moving back toward M'Naghten.

481.   The answer is D. *(Kaplan, ed 5. pp 2118–2120.)* Privileged communication must be provided by statute. Where the privilege exists, it is essentially "owned" by the person whose medical information is being sought. Persons may waive the privilege and allow their psychiatrists to testify. Because there are many qualifications to statutory privilege, some feel that the concept is almost meaningless.

482.   The answer is B. *(Kaplan, ed 5. p 2063.)* In 1860, Elizabeth Packard was confined involuntarily in accordance with an Illinois statute permitting commitment of a married woman on the petition of her husband "without the evidence of insanity or distraction usually required in other cases." Following her release and attempted reconfinement, Mrs. Packard went on a crusade against civil commitment, and her book *Modern Persecution, or Insane Hospitals Unveiled* resulted in the revision of commitment statutes in many states. Jury trials often were mandated as a due-process requirement. However, by the beginning of the twentieth century many of these revised statutes had been repealed. In the 1960s, there was a resurgence of attention concerning the civil rights and abuse of state hospital patients, which has resulted in the current revision of commitment statutes, including greater legal safeguards for persons facing commitment.

483.   The answer is D. *(Michels, vol 3, chap 31, pp 13–16.)* The Tarasoff decision was a landmark case in determining that psychotherapists have an obligation to warn third parties who are in danger. In this instance, the therapist had an obligation to warn the potential victim of a student who had threatened to kill the girl who had rejected him. He ultimately killed her, and thus began the litigation.

484–485.   The answers are: 484-B, 485-A. *(Kaplan, ed 5. p 2114.)* Persons have the right to bequeath their estates to any persons or institutions of their choice. However, for their last will and testament to be valid, they must have testamentary capacity. There is no requirement that they be free of the diagnosis of psychiatric disorder, but testamentary capacity does involve several important criteria. Testators must know who their relatives are and who may have claim to their estate. They must have a reasonable estimate of the extent of their assets. They must know they are signing a will and understand the meaning of that act. Undue influence may be grounds for invalidating part or all of a will if it can be shown that the influence was sufficient to lead the testator to make decisions he or she might not otherwise make. Undue influence relates to voluntariness rather than cognitive capacity and is a distinct and important concept in evaluating a will.

486. The answer is B (1, 3). *(Michels, vol 3, chap 29, p 8.)* There is no legal obligation to accept any patient for therapy, but once the doctor-patient relationship is established, there are legal and ethical obligations on the doctor to keep properly informed about the patient's condition and to provide for psychiatric needs. Abandonment that results in injury may establish grounds for malpractice. The safety and welfare of the patient are paramount. There is an obligation to offer assistance in finding alternative treatment. To simply provide medication does not take into account that the patient may decompensate and injure himself during the period it takes to do this. The therapist might terminate treatment with an uncooperative patient, but only if assistance is given in finding a new therapist.

487. The answer is E (all). *(Talbott, p 1089.)* Issues of informed consent arise whenever any treatment is to be initiated, as well as when there is possible participation in a research study. The ethical issue of "knowing consent" requires that the patient be competent and capable of rationally understanding the relevant issues. The circumstances of the treatment or research must be fully explained, and the patient must voluntarily agree. There must not be coercion or improper inducement. The ethical requirements become particularly important, and difficult, when dealing with psychotic or organically impaired patients whose capacity to evaluate the issues may be clouded.

488. The answer is E (all). *(Michels, vol 3, chap 30, pp 2–7.)* Informed consent is a matter of both ethics and law. It reflects respect for the patient's autonomy as a person who can reason and make decisions regarding personal welfare. The courts have upheld these principles, and it is important that physicians know the laws that govern disclosure in their state. Federal grants in support of research carry very explicit requirements regarding informed consent.

489. The answer is B (1, 3). *(Halleck, pp 89–96. Michels, vol 3, chap 30, pp 6–7.)* While there are many legal debates about just what constitutes an emergency, the courts have generally held that emergencies that threaten life or serious harm to self or others constitute an exception to the requirements for informed consent. Most courts have also rejected the idea that commitment and incompetency are synonymous, and of course not all manifestly psychotic patients are incompetent. The physician need not give information to those patients who waive their rights, but the waiver should be clearly documented in the record.

490. The answer is C (2, 4). *(Michels, vol 3, chap 31, pp 14–16.)* Tarasoff I held that psychotherapists and the police have a duty to warn third parties who are in danger. Tarasoff II stated that once a therapist determines or reasonably should have determined that a patient poses a serious danger of violence to others, he "bears a duty to exercise reasonable care to protect the foreseeable victim of that danger." This is an expansion of the more narrow duty to warn. It leaves unclear what actions would be legally sufficient. The decision also eliminated the police from liability. In 1980 in *Thompson v. County of Alameda* (614 P.2d 728), the California Supreme Court suggested that a "precondition to liability" is an intended victim who is "readily identifiable." Other jurisdictions have gone beyond California and held that an expanded duty exists to groups or categories of potential victims (*Lipari v. Sears, Roebuck & Co.*, 497 Fed Supp. 185 [1980]; *Petersen v. State*, 671 P.2d 230 [1983]).

491.   The answer is C (2, 4). *(Kaplan, ed 5. pp 2121-2122.)* Following the insanity verdict in M'Naghten's case, the outraged Queen and House of Lords demanded from the judges a standard for criminal responsibility. This standard, which did not affect M'Naghten's case, stated that "it must be clearly proved that at the time of the commiting of the act, the party accused was labouring under such a defect of reason, from disease of the mind, as not to know the nature and quality of the act he was doing; or if he did know it, that he did not know that he was doing what was wrong." The defense relied heavily on the ideas of the American psychiatrist Isaac Ray, whose historic work, *A Treatist on the Medical Jurisprudence of Insanity*, was published in 1837. M'Naghten was detained in an asylum for his remaining 22 years. Recently, release of those found not guilty by reason of insanity has occurred more rapidly, and a number of states now place the burden of proof on the state to show the need for continued confinement.

492.   The answer is A (1, 2, 3). *(Kaplan, ed 5. pp 1317-1318, 2121-2122, 2127-2128.)* There are a number of exceptions to the informed consent doctrine. Physicians have a duty to disclose all significant or material risks. They must disclose alternative treatments. Medical emergencies (e.g., when a person is unconscious or otherwise incapable of consenting) have long been accepted as exceptions under the doctrine of implied consent. Courts have also recognized that a person's mental and emotional condition must be taken into account and that discretion must be employed in the manner and style of disclosing information. While there is a degree of latitude for the physician, it is better to err on the side of disclosure. The possibility that disclosure might prompt a person to forgo treatment is not sufficient grounds for withholding information.

493.   The answer is C (2, 4). *(Kaplan, ed 5. pp 2120-2121.)* In establishing a standard for competency of a defendant to stand trial, the U.S. Supreme Court (*Dusky v. United States*, 1960) said that the defendant must have "sufficient present ability to consult with his lawyer with a reasonable degree of rational understanding" and must have "a rational as well as factual understanding of the proceedings against him." The standard is variable in its interpretation, so that a person could be sufficiently rational to be deemed competent to stand trial for trespassing yet incompetent for a complicated murder or embezzlement charge. Competency to stand trial has nothing to do with the defendant's state of mind at the time of the

alleged crime. An accused person's claim of being unable to remember or reconstruct events has met with little sympathetic response from the courts; because
amnesia is not objectively verifiable, judges fear this condition could become "pan-
demic" if it were accepted as a standard for incompetence.

494. The answer is E (all). *(Talbott, pp 1087-1088.)* In "The Principles of Medical Ethics with Annotations Especially Applicable to Psychiatry," the American
Psychiatric Association unequivocally states that sexual activity with patients is
unethical. The intensity of the therapeutic relationship may activate sexual feelings
and fantasies in both patient and therapist; sexual activity has been considered a
dramatic example of the misuse and exploitation of the transference relationship.
Psychiatrists have been prosecuted for rape in a few situations, and this approach
has been advocated by Masters and Johnson. The number of malpractice suits has
been increasing, with substantial settlements and subsequent loss of licensure. Peer
review mechanisms have been of little help in controlling this problem.

495. The answer is A (1, 2, 3). *(Kaplan, ed 5. pp 2108-2109, 2122-2123.)* In
contrast to other witnesses, expert witnesses may give opinion testimony if they
qualify as an expert in the area under consideration. Psychiatrists may give opinions
regarding ultimate issues, such as competence or insanity. They also may use a
variety of tests as a basis for their opinion. In situations in which legally inadmissible
tests are used, the jury is instructed to weigh that evidence only for evaluating the
credibility of the expert's opinion and not for the accuracy of the test. Clear and
convincing evidence, preponderance of the evidence, and proof beyond a reasonable
doubt all are legal standards of proof that judges and juries must use in decision-
making. Expert medical testimony must conform to a "reasonable medical
certainty" standard.

496-500. The answers are: 496-E, 497-A, 498-D, 499-C, 500-C. *(Halleck,
214-219. Michels, vol 3, chap 27, pp 6-9.)* The AMA has recommended, and some
states have codified, that the insanity defense be abolished. There is considerable
question as to whether this can be done constitutionally. Such attempts often direct
that the psychiatrist should only testify as to the *mens rea* elements in criminal trials.
This is testimony that addresses the issue of whether the defendant possessed a
criminal intent or state of mind at the time of the crime.

In 1843 Daniel M'Naghten was accused of killing the secretary of the Prime
Minister of Great Britain. He was acquitted on grounds of insanity, and public
outrage led to the development of the M'Naghten test regarding criminal insanity. It
is a test primarily related to cognitive functions. It became the test of insanity in
many jurisdictions in the United States and is still retained by some states.

The Durham rule, a 1954 decision by the District of Columbia Circuit Court,
eliminated the cognitive issues that were associated with the M'Naghten rule, as
well as the concept of irresistible impulse that had expanded it in some jurisdictions

in order to introduce the concept of volitional control over one's behavior. It gave wide latitude to psychiatric testimony. It was rejected n 1972 because there was simply too much variation in psychiatric opinion as to what constituted the "product of mental disease or mental defect."

The Model Penal Code developed by the American Law Institute (ALI) did not attempt to define mental disease or defect, but it did specify that "the terms 'mental disease' or 'defect' do not include an abnormality manifested only by repeated criminal or otherwise antisocial conduct." This reflected the opinion that sociopaths should not be able to evade criminal responsibility for their acts by claiming that their behavior was on the basis of their psychiatric problem.

Most federal circuit courts and approximately 25 states have adopted at least parts of the rule developed by the ALI. The rule has at least some elements of cognitive (M'Naghten) and volitional (irresistible impulse) determinations. However, it is no longer an issue of "all or nothing." The word "appreciate," for example, acknowledges that a psychotic person may "know" right from wrong, but may lack an ability to truly comprehend the substance and consequences of the behavior. Consider the case of a psychotic who knows that murder is morally and legally wrong, but who kills a neighbor while acting under the influence of paranoid delusions and compelling hallucinations.